T0122829

# Priority Challenges for Social and Behavioral Research and Its Modeling

Paul K. Davis, Angela O'Mahony, Timothy R. Gulden,
Osonde A. Osoba, Katharine Sieck

Prepared for the Defense Advanced Research Projects Agency

For more information on this publication, visit www.rand.org/t/RR2208

**Library of Congress Cataloging-in-Publication Data** is available for this publication.
ISBN: 978-0-8330-9995-2

Published by the RAND Corporation, Santa Monica, Calif.
© Copyright 2018 RAND Corporation
**RAND**® is a registered trademark.

*Cover: jolly/stock.adobe.com.*

## Limited Print and Electronic Distribution Rights

This document and trademark(s) contained herein are protected by law. This representation of RAND intellectual property is provided for noncommercial use only. Unauthorized posting of this publication online is prohibited. Permission is given to duplicate this document for personal use only, as long as it is unaltered and complete. Permission is required from RAND to reproduce, or reuse in another form, any of its research documents for commercial use. For information on reprint and linking permissions, please visit www.rand.org/pubs/permissions.

The RAND Corporation is a research organization that develops solutions to public policy challenges to help make communities throughout the world safer and more secure, healthier and more prosperous. RAND is nonprofit, nonpartisan, and committed to the public interest.

RAND's publications do not necessarily reflect the opinions of its research clients and sponsors.

### Support RAND
Make a tax-deductible charitable contribution at
www.rand.org/giving/contribute

www.rand.org

# Preface

The Defense Advanced Research Projects Agency (DARPA) is investing in diverse aspects of social-behavioral research and modeling. This report is part of a study to assist DARPA in defining challenges and prioritizing such investments. Its initial version was a provocative read-ahead for a workshop of prominent researchers. This final version incorporates insights from that workshop and subsequent research. Comments are welcome and should be addressed to the project leaders Paul K. Davis (pdavis@rand.org) and Angela O'Mahony (aomahon1 @rand.org).

The research in this report was sponsored by Dr. Jonathan Pfautz, a program manager in DARPA's Information Innovation Office (I20). The research was conducted within the International Security and Defense Policy and Acquisition and Technology Policy Centers of the RAND National Defense Research Institute, a federally funded research and development center sponsored by the Office of the Secretary of Defense, the Joint Staff, the Unified Combatant Commands, the Navy, the Marine Corps, the defense agencies, and the defense intelligence community.

For more information on the centers, see www.rand.org/nsrd/ndri /centers/ISDP.html and www.rand.org/nsrd/ndri/centers/ATP.html or contact the directors (contact information is provided on the webpage).

# Table of Contents

# Figures

# Tables

# Summary

## Objectives for Social-Behavioral Research and Modeling

In the years ahead, social-behavioral (SB) modeling (i.e., modeling that reflects behavior of individuals and social entities) *should* help us (1) understand certain classes of SB phenomena with national significance; (2) anticipate how those phenomena *may* plausibly unfold; (3) estimate potential desirable and undesirable effects of additional events in the world or of possible U.S. or adversary interventions; and (4) inform decisionmaking. The phenomena of interest span a broad gamut that includes radicalization for terrorism, the weakening of democracy and national cohesion by foreign information operations campaigns, improving prospects for stability after international interventions, managing behaviors of populations after natural disasters, and dealing with opioid or obesity epidemics. Each such topic would be a good "national challenge," as discussed later. Each has complex multi-dimensional social phenomena that are difficult to analyze without the unique power of modeling. In other domains, such modeling helps planners to strategize, plan, design, and adapt. It helps to avoid blunders and bad side effects of policy interventions.

Today's SB modeling and related analysis is contributing far less to the study of such national issues than it could. Major advances are needed. But in what? In this report we summarize the primary current shortcomings and obstacles—some inherent and some due to current methods and practices. *We identified these obstacles through a review of recent trends and previous research in social-behavioral modeling and simulation, and through discussions and one-on-one conversations with leading experts in this area at RAND workshops and other conferences.*

In this report we then identify and discuss steps that deserve priority attention. Some of our suggestions build on earlier studies; some are newer and more radical.

## Inherent Difficulties and Challenges

Social-behavioral (SB) modeling is famously hard. Three reasons merit pondering:

1. *Complex adaptive systems.* Social systems are complex adaptive systems (CAS) that need to be modeled and analyzed accordingly—not with naïve efforts to achieve accurate and narrow predictions, but to achieve broader understanding, recognition of patterns and phases, limited forms of prediction, and results shown as a function of context and other assumptions. Great advances are needed in understanding the states of complex adaptive systems and their phase spaces and in recognizing both instabilities and opportunities for influence.
2. *Wicked problems.* Many social-behavioral issues arise in the form of so-called wicked problems—i.e., problems with no a priori solutions and with stakeholders that do not have stable objective functions. Solutions, if they are found at all, emerge from human interactions.
3. *Structural dynamics.* The very nature of social systems is often structurally dynamic in that structure changes may emerge after interactions and events. This complicates modeling.

The hard problems associated with CAS need not be impossible. It is not a pipe dream to imagine valuable SB modeling at individual, organizational, and societal scales. After all, complex adaptive systems are only chaotic in certain regions of their state spaces. Elsewhere a degree of prediction and influence is possible. We need to recognize when a social system is or is not controllable.

As for problem wickedness, it should often be possible to understand SB phenomena well enough to guide actions that increase the likelihood of good developments and reduce the likelihood of bad ones. Consider how experienced negotiators can facilitate eventual agreements between nations, or between companies and unions, even when emotions run high and no agreement exists initially about endpoints. Experience helps, and model-based analysis can help to anticipate possibilities and design strategies. Given modern science and technology, opportunities for breakthroughs exist, but they will not come easily.

## Obstacles Due to Shortcomings of Current Practice

### Fragmented Science

To improve SB modeling, we need to understand obstacles, beginning with shortcomings of the science that should underlie it. Current SB theories are many, rich, and informative, but also narrow and fragmented. They do not provide the basis for systemic SB modeling. More nearly comprehensive and coherent theories are needed, but current disciplinary norms and incentives favor continued narrowness and fragmentation. No ultimate "grand theory" is plausible, but a good deal of unification is possible with various domains.

Advances will require more interdisciplinary work at multiple levels of resolution and scales. This is especially demanding because resolution varies along numerous dimensions. Objects of modeling may be individuals or aggregate groups, but different resolutions also exist for spatial and temporal matters, for the attributes ascribed to the objects, and for the interactions among objects. To illustrate, a superficially detailed model may represent millions of individuals but with behaviors driven by simplistic notions of materialistic rational-actor choices. Another model may focus on only a few individuals, but include nuanced information about their attributes. In the practice of modeling and analysis, inconsistencies in scale or levels of analysis are often appropriate because not all detail is comparably relevant. Furthermore, model simplifications are essential for many reasons. Understanding when and how to simplify, however, is not yet well understood in SB modeling.

## Inadequate Comprehensibility, Reviewability, and Reproducibility

A crisis in science has been recognized in recent years. Many published science studies have not been successfully reproduced when (all too rarely) efforts to do so have been attempted. The reasons vary across the sciences, but the result is sobering. Less appreciated is that models and model-based results are frequently incomprehensible and thereby unreviewable. Today's model-based work, especially simulation modeling, is represented in computer code that is often opaque to anyone other than the coder. These problems of comprehensibility, reviewability, and reproducibility impede scientific advances.

## Modeling That Does Not Represent the Science Well

Models represent theories and, in ordinary language, "theory" and "model" are often used interchangeably. The appropriate type of model depends on what is being represented and what questions are being asked. Nonetheless, some general observations on appropriate models apply:

- *Causal, uncertainty-sensitive models.* To represent social-behavioral theory requires increased emphasis on causal models (rather than statistical models) and on uncertainty-sensitive models that routinely display results parametrically in the multiple dimensions that define context. That is, we need models that help us with causal reasoning under uncertainty.
- *Models reflecting subtleties.* Models need to represent subtleties of the science associated with complexity, variable structure, and alternative perspectives (e.g., those of the economist and anthropologist). Some of the subtleties are emergent properties, not something to be "baked in."
- *Relationships.* Many types and formalisms of models are needed, but we need to know how they relate to each other—by analogy, think of tracing the path between quantum statistical physics to classical thermodynamics and engineering formulas.

Current modeling falls short on all of these criteria.

### The Need for Modularity and Composition

To move beyond fragmentation, it is necessary to compose complicated models from lower-level modules. The compositions, however, must be valid for the purpose intended, which can be difficult because the component modules may be based on subtly different assumptions.

Meaningful model compositions are necessary for representing real-world systems, which are often nearly hierarchical or modularly networked. The goal, however, should not be monolithic, officially blessed model federations and databases, but rather the ability to compose appropriately for a given purpose and context while representing uncertainty and disagreement and encouraging competition. For such fit-for-purpose composition to be feasible, community libraries of well-reviewed modules are needed. Competitive and complementary modules will be needed because science is unsettled and different perspectives are needed. Winnowing is good, but over-standardization is a threat. Standing standardized federations are likely to be quite problematic.

### A Myopic View of Model Validity

An obstacle to progress has been an overly narrow view of model validity. *We recommend discussing validity for a specified context along five dimensions: description, explanation, postdiction, exploration and coarse prediction, and classic prediction.*

These distinctions need to be made routinely by researchers, analysts, and consumers of model-based analysis. Few SB models will be valid for classic prediction (accurate, precise, and unequivocal), but much higher aspirations are possible for the other purposes. In contradiction of conventional wisdom, those "other" dimensions of validity are crucial in the progress of science generally. The common focus on prediction when discussing validity is misplaced.

## Strategy for Moving Ahead

### Overview: A Problem-Focused Approach with Multiple Elements

Figure S.1 suggests a way ahead. It highlights (right box) three pillars of progress in social science: theories and modeling, empirical observation

**Figure S.1**
**The Ecology to Respond to National Challenges**

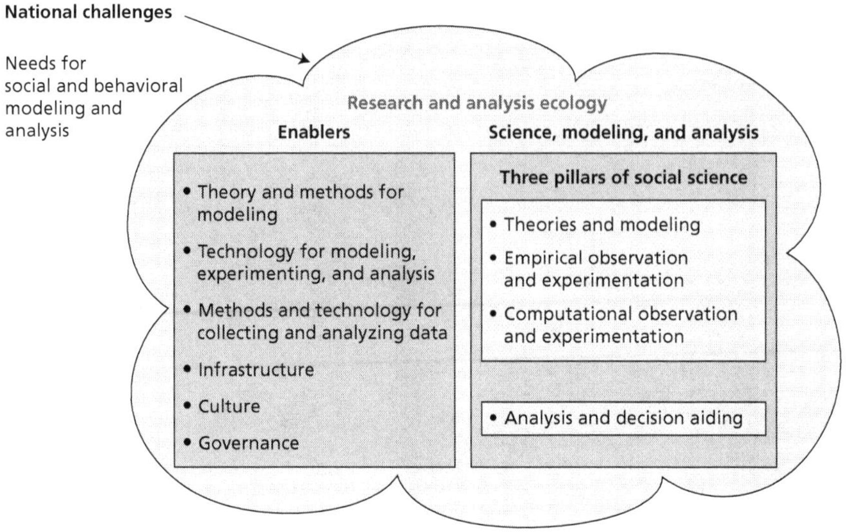

RAND *RR2208-S.1*

and experimentation, and the newer pillar of computational observation and experimentation. Activity occurs in a larger ecology of enabling activities (left side). We suggest that the first step in a strategy for moving forward should be defining a few difficult national challenge problems for multiyear efforts *forcing* interdisciplinary work and providing the concrete context that motivates problem solving. Unlike grand challenges that pose a single crisp technological feat (e.g., long-distance operation of an autonomous road vehicle), these would have subchallenges: (1) tightening links among theory, modeling, and experimentation; (2) seeking better and more unifying theories while retaining alternative perspectives and narratives; (3) challenging experimenters to find new theory-informed ways to obtain relevant information and analyze data; (4) improving methods for using models to inform decisions; (5) challenging theorists and technologists to provide new methods and tools; and (6) nurturing the overall ecology. We discuss those six items in the next paragraphs.

### Tightening the Theory-Modeling-Experimentation Research Cycle

A major issue is how to improve interactions among SB scientists, on the one hand, and "modelers" on the other. The problem is implied by the form of the previous sentence, which distinguishes between scientists and modelers. Why are they distinct whereas in many other fields they often are not? Physicists, engineers, and economists often do their own modeling. Indeed, many social scientists do their own modeling (especially statistical modeling). SB simulation, however, tends to be done by modelers other than social scientists.

A related challenge is improving the degree to which theories and models can be comprehended, reproduced, peer-reviewed, debated, and iterated.

Figure S.2 denotes an idealized way of relating the real and model worlds. It stems from a scientific realism perspective but can address constructivist ideas. It anticipates that knowledge building will involve a combination of induction, deduction, and abduction. The imagery is that a real system exists (the social system of interest, item 1). Real-world observation and experimentation (item 2) help in forming hypotheses about the system's elements, relationships, and processes. Because theory and modeling are always simplifications, we must have particular objectives in mind when asking about the real world or how to model it. We may construct one or more rough-cut system theories in our heads to describe the relevant reality (item 3). Often, alternative notions about the system exist, reflecting different hypotheses, perspectives, or both. This is symbolized by the stacking of icons.

Moving rightward, we construct *coherent* conceptual models of the system (item 4)—including aspects that are important but not observable directly. The conceptual models may be combinations of essays, listings of objects and attributes, or such qualitative devices as influence, stock-and-flow, or network diagrams. The next step, when feasible, is to develop a formal model (item 5), one that specifies all the information needed for computation of model consequences. That is, a specified model must have tight definitions, equations, algorithms, or tables.

In this idealized image rooted in classic pedagogy, the formal model is independent of programming language or is expressed in a high-level language that is easily comprehended by nonprogrammers (i.e., in a

Figure S.2
**An Idealized System View of Theory, Modeling, and Experimentation**

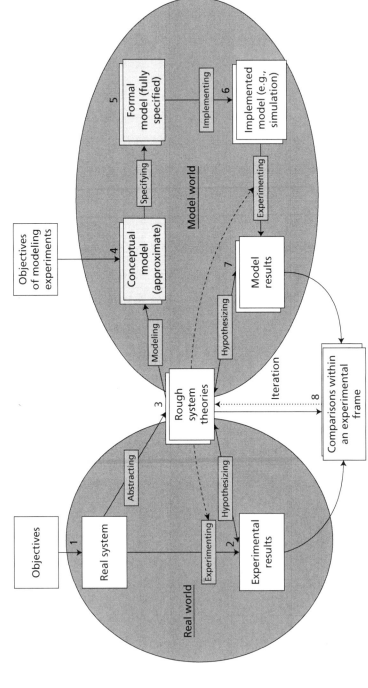

NOTE: Currently, the yellow items (conceptual and formal models) seldom exist separately.

**RAND** *RR2208-S.2*

week rather than a month). The intent is to lay bare the essence of the model without the mind-muddling complications of most computer code and to permit replication, peer review, debate, and iteration. *After* those occur, a formal model can (moving downward) be implemented in other programming languages as convenient (item 6). Moving leftward, the implemented model can then be used with an experimental design to generate model results across the n-dimensional space of model inputs. Results of these exploratory computational experiments (item 7) may falsify, enrich, or support earlier beliefs. For example, they may suggest that the system will show troublesome behavior in certain circumstances not previously considered. Such coarse computational predictions should be compared to experimental results from the real system (item 8). To do so sensibly requires defining the relevant "experimental frame"—i.e., specifying the conditions under which the real and model systems are to be observed and how model results are being used. A model can be considered valid for a particular application in a particular context if the result of using the model's outputs are believed—using all available knowledge—to be adequately close to the result of using the real system's behavior for that experimental frame. The cycle continues (dotted arrow). Overall, Figure S.2 is a virtuous research cycle with a holistic view in which theory, models, empirical inquiry, and computational inquiry are all part of a closely networked system. What follows describes suggested priorities for improving other aspects of the science, theories, models, and larger ecosystem.

### Improving Theory and Related Modeling

Some priorities for SB research are as follows, expressed as objectives at the *functional level*.

1. *Move modeling farther into the science itself.* An example might be an anthropologist professor and graduate student doing the modeling directly or accomplishing this with exceptionally tight teaming across departments. All concerned would be intimately familiar with the conceptual and formal models. This contrasts with a modeler first building a model and only then, annoyingly, calling on social scientists to estimate input values.

2.  *Put a premium on causal models* that include all important variables, whether or not "soft." Ensure that models are faithful to the emerging theory, including allowing system characteristics to be emergent. As part of this objective, develop methods for variable-structure simulation to include versions in which changes are emergent.

3.  *Define context.* Go beyond hand-waving reference to "it all depends on context" by defining what characterizes context— e.g., state variables, exogenous events, and aspects of history.

4.  *Build in uncertainty analysis from the outset.* Build uncertainties about model structure as well as model-parameter values into the very fabric of models. Prepare for analysis under deep uncertainty.

5.  *Use portfolios of analytic tools.* The portfolio should include simulation but also, for example, equilibrium models, static models applicable at a point in time, knowledge-based simulation, qualitative models, and such human-in-the-loop mechanisms as games and interactive simulation laboratories.

6.  *Seek multiresolution, multiperspective families of models* that cut across levels of detail and perspective (e.g., across individual, local, regional, and more global population levels, or across immediate and longer-term time scales). Partly this will involve respecting different views of phenomena, including culture-sensitive views.

7.  *Synthesize across theories*, where feasible. A unifying theory may, for example, explain that a behavior can be due to any one or a combination of pathways depending on circumstances and history.

8.  *Translate across theories.* Sharpen understanding of where useful theories are equivalent but expressed in different languages or formalisms, and where they are inherently incommensurate (e.g., individual-centric and culture-centric models).

9.  *Design for good practice.* Design for reproducibility, comprehensibility, peer review, and iteration.

10. *Organize for interdisciplinary work* that is both collaborative and competitive.

**Improving Computational and Empirical Experimentation**

A somewhat shorter list of admonitions applies to improving the data obtained from real-world experiments and computational experimentation.

1.  *Seek the right data even if inconvenient.* Ensure that empirical data are appropriate for the purpose (i.e., the national challenge). In particular, address difficult-to-measure and sometimes latent qualitative variables, seeking representative albeit uncertain data rather than poor proxies.
2.  *Exploit opportunities.* Better yet, exploit modern and emerging data sources, which are sometimes massive, sometimes sparse, and often riddled with correlations and biases.
3.  *Shorten the cycle.* Greatly increase the speed with which needed data can be obtained and processed.
4.  *Give nontrivial multivariate theory a chance.* Use theory-informed approaches wherever possible when designing and conducting empirical or computational experiments. These approaches should not be theory-*imposing*, but they should stress testing and enriching theories (multivariate, causal system theories, not simple hypotheses or correlations). Healthy competition should exist between data-driven and theory-informed work.
5.  *Use exploratory analysis.* Analyze computational data with the methods of exploratory analysis, looking, for example, at outcome landscapes (region plots) and phase diagrams rather than point outcomes.

**Improving Methods and Technology for Modeling and Experimentation**

The priorities expressed above assume methods and technology for modeling, data collection, and analysis. Some of what is needed does not yet exist. Some questions should be priorities for providers of modeling theory, methods, and tools. *How do we*:

- Build into models the capacity for routine multidimensional deep-uncertainty analysis?

- Build variable-structure simulations in which agent types, the character of their reasoning, and their parameters change or even emerge within the course of simulation?
- Define the suite (portfolio) of methods and tools needed to represent and compare different scales and alternative models with different narratives or perspectives? How do they relate?
- Conduct theory-informed empirical and computational experiments? How do we design, collect, and analyze?
- Make the best use of modern data sources, which are sometimes massive, sometimes sparse, and often riddled with subtle correlations?
- Infer causal relations from only partially controlled observational data?
- Accomplish *heterogeneous* fusion and otherwise "manage knowledge" so that information can be used despite variations of scale, formalism, and character?
- Build conceptual and formal models that are comprehensible to subject-area scientists and subject to reproducibility, peer review, debate, sharing, and iteration?
- Reconceive "composability" to include accommodating analysis under multidimensional deep uncertainty and improving comprehensibility and the ability to check composition validity for context (testing fitness for purpose)?
- Communicate with decisionmakers using cognitively effective mechanisms?

## Modernizing Model-Based Decision Aiding

Great strides have been made over the last 25 years related to model-based analysis for complex problems, and some of the corresponding lessons need to be assimilated in conceiving and nurturing research on SB modeling. These have implications for the building and testing of models, design and conduct of analysis, and communication of insights to decisionmakers. The most important, arguably, have to do with planning under deep uncertainty. The modern approach requires a shift of analytic paradigm: Instead of attempting to optimize some outcome (subject to many dubious assumptions), the preferred strategy is one that will do "adequately" across the range of reasonable assumptions that constitute deep uncertainty. That is, one seeks strategies that are flexible, adaptive, and robust (i.e., that will accommodate changes in an objective or goal, that will accommodate unexpected circumstances, and that will deal adequately with initial shocks). Again, embracing this paradigm requires changing the way in which we build and use models.

## Attending to Culture, Governance, and Other Ecosystem Issues

Although the items that follow are less about research than about management issues for government, we include them because the overall effort needs to address all aspects of the challenge's ecostructure.

### Cultural Mindsets

Mismatches currently exist—among both recipients of research and the researchers themselves—between what is sought and what should be sought in describing knowledge and informing reasoned decisionmaking. Mindset changes are needed as indicated in Table S.1, especially

**Table S.1**
**Cultural Mindset Changes**

| From | To |
|---|---|
| Seeking narrow point predictions and optimization (akin to engineering) | Seeking analysis of wicked problems and development of robust strategies |
| Seeking a simple once-and-for-all strategy | Seeking explicitly adaptive strategies that require routine monitoring and adjustment |
| Seeking "human terrain" with solid, fixed data | Seeing the "terrain" as complex, heterogeneous, and dynamic—in structure, not just attribute values |
| Predicting and acting | Exploring and proceeding with adaptation expected |
| Using unvalidated models or generically validated models to inform particular important decisions | Deemphasizing "generic" validation and elevating the importance of analysis-specific validation |
| Receiving and acting on model-generated answers | Interacting with models (including games) to understand systems and phenomena, including relationships, possibilities, and corresponding adaptations |

in the domain of SB issues. These changes would be consistent with modern research in the decision sciences.

### Infrastructure

The relevant elements of infrastructure include vigorous academic and private-world research programs in the United States and other countries, related funding, and mechanisms for interaction. Infrastructure includes laws, regulations, funding strategies, and relationships that encourage balances among, for example, openness, sharing, and protection of intellectual property and privacy rights (see below).

### Governance and Ethics

One class of issues involves the ethics of ensuring privacy and respect for civil liberties. Many elements of research will involve data collection and data analysis, some of which could cause difficulties and, in some instances, violate the intentions of law. It is critical to maintain and help establish the highest standards on such matters, but to do so will require continued analysis and innovation and perhaps promulgation of suitable laws. A second set of issues involves ensuring that model-based insights do not have unanticipated and seriously negative side effects when applied to the real world.

### Social-Behavioral Laboratories as a Mechanism

One mechanism for proceeding is to have, for each national challenge, a virtual social-behavioral modeling laboratory (SBML). This might be seen merely as an organized program akin to the Human Genome Project of years past, but we use the term "laboratory" to convey a sense of purposeful and organized scientific inquiry to "crack" a particular challenge.

An SBML (Figure S.3) would exist for five to ten years and would enable interdisciplinary sharing and synergism. An SBML approach would *not* seek a monolithic standardized model federation with approved structure and databases. Instead, the approach would be dynamic and iterative with routine competition, iteration, and evolution. Meaningful model compositions would be constructed for specific purposes. The SBML activities would include both simulation modeling (generating system behavior over time) and other forms of qualitative and quantitative modeling, including participative modeling and

## Figure S.3
## An SBML for a Particular National Challenge

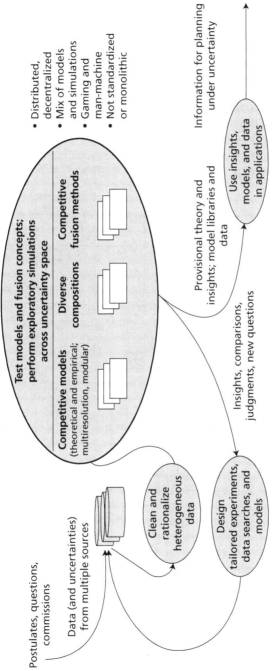

other forms of human interaction such as gaming. Related conferences would focus on the national challenge, the state of related social science, the degree to which modeling and simulation (M&S) represent that science, the products of empirical work and computational experimentation, and how to characterize knowledge and inform decisions. Comparing lessons from multiple national challenges would reveal further generalizations.

To end on a philosophical note, a successful SBML approach would foster a new "epistemic culture" in social-behavioral research: Those participating would be building knowledge in a different and more multifaceted way than is customary. The result might reflect not just scientific knowledge and craft but also what Aristotle called *phronesis* (practical wisdom and thoughtfulness, reflecting an understanding of ethics, and situational subtleties). The word may be Greek, but the ideas endure.

# Acknowledgments

We thank the many participants in the DARPA-sponsored workshops held by RAND in Washington, D.C., on December 9, 2016, and in Santa Monica, California, on April 3–4, 2017. The earlier workshop addressed issues of privacy and ethics in social-behavioral research; the later and much larger workshop dealt with social-behavioral research and its modeling. Before and after the workshops we benefited in particular from lengthy discussions with Robert Axtel, Chris Glazner, Levent Yilmaz, Cory Lofdahl, Bill Rouse, and Andreas Tolk. We greatly benefited from comments on the draft report by Laura McNamara (Sandia) and by RAND colleagues Thomas Szayna, Seth Jones, Ed Balkovich, and Aaron Frank. A version of the report's summary was presented as a paper at the 2017 meeting of the Computational Social Science Society, the peer reviewers for which provided helpful comments. The entire study benefited from extensive discussion at the outset with Jonathan Pfautz (DARPA).

# CHAPTER ONE

# Introduction

## Objectives

This report documents an effort to assist DARPA in identifying priorities as it invests in social-behavioral (SB) research and related modeling.[1] Priority setting depends on objectives. In this report we have in mind that, in the long run, SB modeling and related analysis should help:

1. Understand certain SB phenomena of national importance—such diverse examples as violent extremism, threats to the United States from information warfare attacks, public response to natural disasters, and population health problems generally.
2. Anticipate how those phenomena may unfold.
3. Estimate potential direct and indirect effects from events that may occur naturally, from actions of adversary nations or groups, or from actions of U.S. federal, state, or local governments.
4. Provide *useful* aids to planning under uncertainty, including the deep uncertainties that often arise when dealing with human and social phenomena.

Modeling and simulation—if well rooted in social-behavioral science—can, along with ubiquitous data and data analytics—materially inform

---

[1] We refer to social-behavioral (SB) research without distinguishing between S and B. Scholarly distinctions are inconsistent, and some disciplines cross boundaries (e.g., sociology, anthropology, social psychology, and behavioral economics).

planning about some of the most vexing national problems of our day. Unfortunately, the current state of social-behavioral modeling and related analysis is not yet up to the job. There have been some successes but nothing close to the potential.

To be sure, non-modeling social science methods (e.g., trend analyses, discovery of statistical correlations, field surveys, psychological experimentation) already contribute to decisionmaking. Consider the impact of SB science and data analytics on commercial marketing and political campaigns (Nickerson and Rogers, 2014; Issenberg, 2012; Confessore and Hakim, 2017). Consider the rise of behavioral economics and "nudge policies" (Perry et al., 2015; Sunstein, 2014; Thaler and Sunstein, 2009), the value of psychology in understanding the political chasm in modern America (Haidt, 2013), or the threat posed to democracies by foreign influence operations that exploit social divisions (Waltzman, 2017). These methods, however, have significant shortcomings. Computer modeling, which includes simulation and human-in-the-loop simulation, has long been recognized as having great potential for addressing those shortcomings.[2]

It is easy to be skeptical given the notoriously difficult nature of social-behavioral phenomena, but glimpses of the potential can be seen from past efforts. Epidemiological modeling has long assisted the Centers for Disease Control (CDC) in detecting and understanding epidemics early enough to intervene effectively (Hethcote, 2000; Homer and Hirsch, 2006). Vision models, such as feature integration, exploit information from both cognitive psychology and neuroscience and have proved highly successful (Quinlan, 2003). System dynamics modeling has been applied in many ways over the decades, sometimes representing behavioral considerations to some degree. Agent-based modeling (ABM) is still relatively new, but has been used for some years at Argonne National Laboratories to work with diverse stakeholders in simulating and understanding the operation of complex power systems at the core

---

[2]  Visions of the system-dynamics variety can be seen in, for example, Forrester, 1969, and Dörner, 1997. Scott Page of the University of Michigan has an online course that gives strong reasons for modeling; see http://www.youtube.com/watch?v=8InQk0-PmPc. Page emphasizes the value of models for deciding, strategizing, and designing.

of national infrastructure (North and Macal, 2007). It has also been used in economic modeling of power systems (Tesfatsion, 2018). An early version of ABM was used at RAND in Cold War game-structured simulation to understand the dynamics of nuclear escalation and de-escalation (National Research Council, 2014, pp. 73–77). ABM and other modeling has also been used to advise top executives of health care organizations and commercial companies.[3] From these examples we conclude that it is no pipe dream to imagine that SB models can achieve the objectives identified above. Nonetheless, we and past studies have concluded that SB models are not yet even close to achieving their potential, especially for the kinds of national-level policy challenges mentioned previously.

*Our objectives, then, include diagnosing the problems, identifying challenges, and recommending ways to move ahead so that SB modeling will be more powerfully useful for aiding decisionmaking. Many reasons exist to be bullish about breakthroughs ahead, but they will not come easily.*

## Background

The background for our report is that DARPA tasked us to conduct a study to help identify challenges and priorities for research in social-behavioral modeling, primarily with complex systems in mind. DARPA was anticipating investing in a several related programs in 2017 and beyond (several programs have subsequently been started). The project would reach out to numerous respected figures in the research community, in part by conducting workshops to elicit a sense of the current state of the art in social-behavioral modeling and a sense of what should come next. This report is not workshop proceedings but rather our effort to pull findings together. An earlier draft was used as a serious-strawman read-ahead for participants in a two-day workshop held April 3–4, 2017, in Santa Monica, California. The current report also draws on results of an earlier workshop dealing with ethics

---

[3]   See examples at www.systemdynamics.org. See also Rouse and Boff, 2005; Rouse, 2015, which describes the use of multiple model formalisms; and Youngman and Hadzikadic, 2014.

and privacy issues, which was held on December 9, 2016, in RAND's Arlington, Virginia, office. This final version reflects lessons learned from the workshops and our post-workshop research. Thus it has benefited from the work and suggestions of many researchers, but is solely our responsibility.

Our project built on foundations of past work, such as indicated in Table 1.1. These earlier foundational efforts provided an excellent overview of the breadth and objectives of previous SB modeling. Most, however, had taken place quite some time ago. Given such background, we focused our own work primarily on recent developments, on framing current issues, and on encouraging a shift away from discussion of difficulties (common in earlier workshops and conferences) toward ambitious next steps. DARPA's intent was for our project and report to help in *moving on*. Before proceeding, however, let us comment briefly on the first two reports of Table 1.1, which were especially helpful.

A decade ago, the National Research Council (NRC) conducted a comprehensive three-year study. The *2008 NRC Report*'s recommendation was to develop the infrastructure to promote and sustain collaborative advances in SB modeling to increase its utility for decisionmaking. This report and DARPA's new investments are in some respects a belated follow-up to that guidance. Table 1.2 summarizes the NRC study's conclusions and recommendations briefly. The final chapter in that report was particularly helpful. Regrettably, DoD had not followed up on that report very well because of intervening priorities related to the war efforts in Iraq and Afghanistan. Thus, a good deal of catching up would be necessary.

A report by the Sandia National Laboratories, the *2011 Sandia Workshop*, was sponsored by the Defense Threat Reduction Agency (DTRA). It featured discussion and soul-searching on computational modeling and simulation (McNamara et al., 2011). Figure 1.1 is adapted from that report and suggests that computational social science should be understood and evaluated separately for its contributions to social science, computational science, and analysis for decision support. That is, the activity is contributing to three domains, and a given example of computational modeling may contribute well for one but not for the

**Table 1.1**
**A Baseline of Past Summary Discussions**

| Publisher | Authors/Chairs | Book or Report Title | Citation |
|---|---|---|---|
| National Research Council (NRC) | Zacharias, MacMillan, and Van Hemel | Behavioral Modeling and Simulation: From Individuals to Societies | Zacharias et al., 2008 |
| Sandia National Laboratories | McNamara, Trucano, and Gieseler | Challenges in Computational Social Modeling and Simulation for National Security Decision-Making | McNamara et al., 2011 |
| Springer Publications | Kött and Citrenbaum | Estimating Impact: A Handbook of Computational Methods and Models for Anticipating Economic, Social, Political and Security Effects in International Interventions | Kött and Citrenbaum, 2010 |
| MITRE | Egeth, Klein, and Schmorrow | Sociocultural Behavior Sensemaking: State of the Art in Understanding the Operational Environment | Egeth et al., 2014 |
| NRC | Keller-McNulty | Defense Modeling, Simulation, and Analysis: Meeting the Challenge | National Research Council, 2006 |
| NRC | Standing Committee on Technology Insight—Gauge, Evaluate, and Review (TIGER) | The Rise of Games and High-Performance Computing for Modeling and Simulation | National Research Council, 2010 |
| NRC | Pool (rapporteur) | Sociocultural Data to Accomplish Department of Defense Missions: Toward a Unified Social Framework: Workshop Summary | National Research Council and Pool, 2011 |
| | Hadzikadic, O'Brien, and Khouja | Managing Complexity: Practical Considerations in the Development and Application of ABMs to Contemporary Policy Challenges | Hadzikadic et al., 2013 |

**Table 1.2**
**Themes from a 2008 NRC Report**

| NRC Results | Items | Elaboration |
| --- | --- | --- |
| Categories of Problem | Modeling strategy: match to real world | Difficulties in this area are created either by inattention to the real world being modeled or by unrealistic expectations about how much of the world can be modeled and how close a match between model and world is feasible. |
| | Verification, validation, and accreditation | These important functions often are made more difficult by expectations that verification, validation, and accreditation (VV&A)—as it has been defined for the validation of models of physical systems—can be usefully applied to individual, organizational, and societal (IOS) models. |
| | Modeling tactics: design internal structure | Problems are sometimes generated by unwarranted assumptions about the nature of the social, organizational, cultural, and individual behavior domains, and sometimes by a failure to deliberately and thoughtfully match the scope of the model to the scope of the phenomena to be modeled. |
| | Physical versus human behavior; uncertainty and adaptation | Problems arise from unrealistic expectations of how much uncertainty reduction is plausible in modeling human and organizational behavior, as well as from poor choices in handling the changing nature of human structures and processes. |
| | Combining components and federating models | Problems arise from the way in which linkages within and across levels of analysis change the nature of system operation. They occur when creating multilevel models and when linking together more specialized models of behavior into a federation of models. |
| Recommendations | Large-scale, integrated, cross-disciplinary programs | |
| | Research in six areas | Theory development (especially low-level social). |

**Table 1.2—Continued**

| NRC Results | Items | Elaboration |
|---|---|---|
| | | Uncertainty, dynamic adaptability, and rational behavior. |
| | | Data collection methods (problem-focused collection, ontologies, standards, massively multiplayer online games [MMOGs]). |
| | | Federated models (across components, levels; semantic interoperability). |
| | | Validation and usefulness. |
| | | Tools and infrastructure for model building. |
| | Multidisciplinary conferences, workshops, etc. | Communication, education, sharing. |

others. This point proved important to us in writing the current report about research priorities.

The Sandia team also concluded that stronger inputs were needed from social scientists, that simulation is not always the best tool, and that computational social science should be seen as a *process* rather than an artifact—i.e., that the greatest benefits may come from the knowledge gained and relationships created during the knowledge-production activity rather than from particular simulation-model results. The workshop report discussed differences between physical and social sciences and recognized that model validation is different and difficult for these domains. All of these conclusions remain valid and are reflected throughout our own report.

The other references mentioned in Table 1.1 are rich with individual chapters on numerous topics; we drew on many of them in the course of writing this report. The Kött-Citrenbaum and Egeth-Klein-Schmorrow books drew on work in DARPA's Conflict, Modeling, Planning, and Outcome Experimentation (COMPOEX) program and the Human, Social and Culture Behavior Modeling (HSCB) program at the Department of Defense (DoD). Shaped by the tactical

**Figure 1.1**
**Seeing Contributions of Computational**
**Social Science as Interdisciplinary**

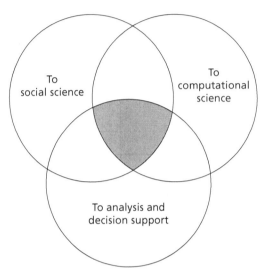

SOURCE: Adapted from McNamara et al., 2011.
RAND *RR2208-1.1*

and operational needs arising in the wars in Iraq and Afghanistan, both programs were rather different in character from most of what we discuss in this report.[4] The Hadzikadic-O'Brien-Khouja book drew on results of another DARPA program, one confronting the relationship between major national and international problems and complex adaptive systems. The program sought "to transform agent-based models into platforms for predicting and evaluating policy responses to challenges" (Hadzikadic et al., 2013, p.12; Youngman and Hadzikadic, 2014).

---

[4]  The COMPOEX program sought "transformational technologies to enhance the capability of military commanders and their civilian leaders to plan and conduct campaigns in a complex operational environment." The HSCB program sought "technologies, tools, and systems to help operations planners, intelligence analysts, operations analysts, and wargames represent, understand, and forecast socio-cultural behavior at the strategic, operational, and tactical level" (Egeth et al., 2014).

**Figure 1.2**
**An Ecology Perspective**

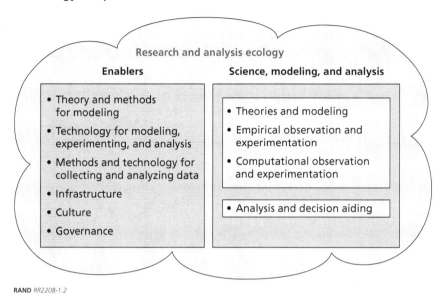

RAND RR2208-1.2

## Structure of Report

In structuring our study and this report we embraced an ecosystem view of the overall area as indicated in Figure 1.2. On the right side, we adopt the three-pillar view of science often urged by computational social scientists (President's Information Technology Advisory Committee, 2005). The pillars of this view are theories and modeling, empirical experimentation, and computational experimentation.[5]

The remainder of this report is structured to assist the process of moving on with this ecostructure in mind. Chapter 3 describes important points that we believe can be agreed upon and stipulated. It also suggests the broad outlines of a strategy. Chapters 4–9 suggest, respectively, ways to improve the overall research cycle; theory and modeling; experimentation; linkages to decision aiding; methods and technology; and infrastructure,

---

[5] Appreciating the role of computational experimentation traces to the work of the Sante Fe Institute in the 1980s and two books in the 1990s (Axelrod, 1997; Epstein and Axtell, 1996).

culture, and governance. The Summary is a more lengthy review of the main text as a whole.

Achieving the objectives outlined previously will depend not just on the three pillars but also on the enablers shown on the left side of Figure 1.2. New theory, methods, and technology are needed just to do the modeling and data work called for on the right. So also, attitudinal and cultural changes will be necessary for reasons elaborated later. Governance might seem an odd item to include in Figure 1.2, but incentives are needed to cause the interdisciplinary work to occur. Further, it is necessary to maintain high ethical standards with respect to privacy and other civil liberties. How to do so, while also encouraging the scientific advances, is a challenge for governance, as discussed in an earlier workshop of this project led by Rebecca Balebako (Balebako et al., 2017).

# CHAPTER TWO

# Difficulties, Challenges, and a Broad Strategy for Next Steps

## Inherent Difficulties of Social-Behavioral Science and Its Modeling

Social sciences and the natural sciences are alike in many ways, more so than is sometimes realized. According to philosopher Susan Haack, a key difference is that much of social science (what she refers to as intentional social science)

> tries to understand people's behavior by coming up with explanatory hypotheses about their beliefs, goals, etc. (Haack, 2011, p. 166)

Haack sees the primary differences between natural and social sciences as lying in the nature of explanations and evidence, which she discusses in Chapter 6 of her work, "The Same, Only Different." She begins her chapter with an apt quotation from Adolf Lowe: "Only if a region of inquiry can be opened up in which both the scientific and the humanist approach play their characteristic roles may we ever hope to gain knowledge of man—knowledge rather than figment, and of man rather than of social atoms."

Some of the challenges for social-behavioral modeling have long been recognized. For example, Herbert Simon introduced the concept of bounded rationality in the 1960s. As he mentioned in his later tome on the subject (Simon, 1957):

> the first consequence of the principle of bounded rationality is that the intended rationality of an actor requires him to construct

a simplified model of the real situation in order to deal with it. He behaves rationally with respect to this model, and such behavior is not even approximately optimal with respect to the real world. To predict his behavior we must understand the way in which this simplified model is constructed, and its construction will certainly be related to his psychological properties as a perceiving, thinking, and learning animal.

In a later well-beloved book, Simon discussed his ideas about artificial intelligence and, significantly, the need to learn from *complex* systems in nature—e.g., human systems with their "nearly decomposable" nature (Simon, 1996). Perhaps responding to Jared Diamond's comment that "soft sciences are often harder than hard sciences" (Diamond, 1987), Simon famously wrote (p. 304):

> The true line is not between "hard" natural science and "soft" social science, but between precise science limited to highly abstract and simple phenomena in the laboratory and inexact science and technology dealing with complex problems in the real world.

Dealing with complex problems in the real world is surely difficult, but that is what makes some of them interesting and "DARPA-hard." We elaborate on the difficulties with three overlapping observations. *Confronting these three matters is at the core of moving forward.*

## Complex Adaptive Systems

Social systems are often complex adaptive systems (CAS), the study of which has come to the forefront over the last thirty years, albeit with antecedents going back at least to the nineteenth-century mathematician Henri Poincaré. As is now well known, the behavior of such systems can be very difficult to anticipate. Even small changes in initial conditions or events that occur over time can have outsized effects on the system's dynamics. In some circumstances, behavior can even be chaotic.[1]

---

[1]   CAS is well described in many books (Holland, 1998; Holland and Mimnaugh, 1996; Page, 2010; Bar-Yam, 1997). Interestingly, related matters in theoretical chemistry (which does not have sentient agents) were described in the 1970s (Nicolis and Prigogine, 1977).

Despite common impressions to the contrary, this does *not* mean that it is hopeless to study CAS with the hope of making some predictions or exerting some degree of influence or control. Nor does it mean that "nonlinear" implies chaos. It means only that a CAS is uncontrollable in certain of its states. Consider that the excellent steering, braking, and road-handling of modern passenger cars is the result of complex nonlinear controls (nonlinear can be "good"). In some circumstances, however—i.e., for some combinations of speed, acceleration, and road angle—all bets are off. In such a state, a small change may lead to any of markedly different but potentially catastrophic outcomes. The admonition is to avoid getting into those states—i.e., to drive "within the intended envelope."[2] As a social example, consider a vigorous crowd. Will it settle down, divide into separate but peaceful groups, turn into verbal battle among groups, or turn into a chaotic and violent melee? Leaders as diverse as high school principals and politicians know things about how to "influence" crowds and about when efforts to do so may make things worse rather than better.[3] In such cases, closing down activities may be important. More generally, a key issue is recognizing which states are and are not subject to a degree of influence or control. And, for those that are, what can be achieved and with what risks?

### Wicked Problems

A particularly deep issue when addressing social-behavioral phenomena is that associated with so-called wicked problems (i.e., problems with no preordained solution, nor even a priori objectives to be achieved). Instead, people may in the course of interacting come to conclude that they can share some common objectives and cooperate in some strategy. Or they may not. Such developments are not baked in and predictable from game theory or operations research; rather, they *emerge*.[4]

---

[2]   One of us (Davis) was first sensitized to this point from a discussion with Caltech's John Doyle in a 1990s panel study (National Research Council, 1997).

[3]   Some work on such matters has been done from the CAS perspective (Leveror, 2016).

[4]   Horst Rittel introduced the term "wicked problem," which was adapted by Charles Churchman (Churchman, 1967). Wicked problems play prominently in "soft operations research," which has been more popular in Europe than in the United States (Rosenhead and Mingers, 2002).

Recognizing the ubiquity of wicked problems can be profound and unsettling because so much formal education prepares us to recognize and solve non-wicked problems, preferably by finding the optimal solution.

### The Dynamic Character of People and Social Systems

Although modelers traditionally like to define "the system" carefully, the system boundaries are typically fixed (i.e., static). Social systems, however, not only exhibit dynamics but change their structural character and the character of interactions over time. Even value structures change (not just relative weights of pre-existing values). Social scientists sometimes note with dismay how military organizations attach themselves to the concept of "human terrain" and try to characterize it neatly and definitively in cultural databases, even though the characteristics may change markedly, and sometimes quickly.[5]

Having discussed top-level difficulties in social-behavioral research, the next several sections summarize major obstacles to progress. They relate to current disciplinary norms, the nature of the models needed, and synthesis.

## Obstacles Due to Shortcomings of Current Practice

If some obstacles are inherent, others are not. In particular, current disciplinary boundaries, norms, and practices are in some ways obstacles to progress in SB research of interest in this report.

### Fragmentation

A companion paper provides an overview of current social-behavioral theory (Nyblade et al., 2017) and illustrates that it is possible, from a remove, to recognize broad themes in social and behavioral theories that provide considerable unity at an abstract level. This is a partial antidote to the common impression that social-behavioral theories exist in bewilderingly large numbers, but are typically narrow and fragmented. Still,

---

[5]   See McNamara et al., 2011, particularly a background paper by Robert Albro (Albro, 2011).

few efforts are made to seek more general theories that pull together those fragments coherently. Indeed, practitioners are so insistent that "context dominates" as to resist looking for more general theories.

## Methods and Norms

The dominant methods and norms in the social-behavioral sciences are part of the reason for fragmentation. Qualitative researchers do not usually build models, certainly not computational models. Instead, they rely on text and reasoning, perhaps with structuring expressed with tables. Quantitative researchers use empirical methods that measure correlations and test discrete hypotheses. Their research tends to be driven by a disciplinary norm favoring a particular kind of parsimony and regression models with only a few measurable variables and coefficients. It tends to dismiss variables that are "soft" (approximate, qualitative, difficult to measure) and/or variables that appear to have low statistical significance when used to explain empirical data.[6] This practice is troubling to those in other fields that emphasize causal modeling and that retain variables seen to be important, even if the importance is not evident in the available data. After all, to drop a variable is to assume that it is not important (i.e., that it is approximated as 0 in a sum or as 1 in a product).

Such issues have long been debated within portions of the social science community. A few decades ago, quantitative analysis (statistical in nature) was regarded as more scientific, with qualitative research being seen as "lesser." This is no longer the case; today, well-structured qualitative research is highly regarded and, in some quarters, it is statistics-based quantitative analysis that is viewed with skepticism or antipathy. The qualitative and quantitative tribes still exist—with their own conferences, book series, and journals—but a better balance exists and graduate students learn about the strengths and weaknesses of the different approaches.[7]

---

[6] See Forrester, 1963. We note that a variable may have low statistical significance in empirical work because, for example, (1) the proxies used to approximate the variable are poor, (2) there is too little data to prove a valid but small effect, or (3) the variable acts only through nonlinear composite variables.

[7] Although tribalism is a problem, as noted by reviewers and by Lawrence Kuznar (Kuznar, 2008), exceptions exist. One mentioned was the late anthropologist Michael Agar, whose

Some other developments have occurred, but have not disseminated evenly across fields. In economics, for example, great emphasis is now placed on looking for causal relationships and *causal models*, even when the researchers must depend heavily on empirical data that is not the result of controlled experiments, such as in the famous randomly controlled trials of medical research. Econometricians have developed excellent *quasi-experimental methods* that depend on natural experiments that exploit available data in more meaningful ways (Angrist and Pischke, 2009).

Another noteworthy development has been *comparative case studies* as pioneered by Alexander George, who saw case studies as key ingredients in developing theory (George and Bennett, 2005). Even in such work, models tend to be more like tables or logical constructs than the computer models used routinely in many domains. The richness and subtleties of theory tend to be described in text.

All of this is a poor match for the building of computer models to represent social-behavioral theory. So also, statistical data is often a poor fit for connecting to theory.[8] As noted in earlier reviews, the modeling community is not receiving what it needs from the science community (McNamara et al., 2011). Candidly, we also observe that many in the modeling community do not try very hard to get into the scientific subtleties because of being more passionate about the programming than the science.

---

work ranged from linguistics to agent-based modeling, and from fieldwork to mathematical models. He firmly admonished students that scientists need to engage with real people in real settings to understand who they are and what they are trying to do before drawing generalizations (Agar, 2013).

[8]   Related discussion dates back at least to the economist John Maynard Keynes in 1939 (Forrester and Senge, 1996, p. 16). Statistical data are often not suitable for testing or informing causal models. One reason is that an important causal variable may fail a T-test of statistical significance because of measurement-error problems (Forrester and Senge, 1996, p. 17). More important, if a phenomenon depends primarily on a composite variable, a regression in terms of the various $X_i$ might see none of them as important. In the physical sciences, it is common for theory to highlight composite variables such as natural dimensionless ratios. Some authors refer to the importance of using theory to identify "aggregation fragments" (Davis and Bigelow, 1998).

It follows that we see the need for more work on social and behavior theory that is *causal, multivariate, integrative, coherent, and more general* wherever feasible. This does not mean that we harbor notions of some grand overall theory of everything (such a theory does not yet exist even in physics, much less in the human domain where it is likely implausible).[9] Moving in that direction, however, is attractive compared to the current situation.

We elaborate in the following sections, but the improvements in theory that we see as necessary will often be *qualitative* because of the nature of social-behavioral phenomena. So be it. Ideally, hybrid methods are desirable, as when quantitative analysis is strongly informed by more detailed case studies and subsequent case studies are informed by quantitative research.[10]

## Representing the Richness of the Science

In our view, social-behavioral modeling needs to be much more strongly informed in the future by the strongest features of the related science, rather than sometimes settling for what social scientists see as a simplistic gloss.

### *Need for Multivariate Causal Models*

Social-behavioral science makes extensive use of statistical methods, and that will continue for many reasons. For the purposes of the kind of research we discuss in this report, however, a premium exists for *causal* models and for models that deal well with uncertainty. Often, the models needed will be multivariate and sometimes nonlinear (see discussion in Chapter 4). In such cases, the standard social science method of making and testing discrete hypotheses has significant shortcomings, especially when the hypotheses only deal with easy-to-measure

---

[9] Philosopher Nancy Cartwright discusses the need to see science as a patchwork (Cartwright, 1999), as does anthropologist Mel Konner (Konner, 2003). Even so, we believe that within domains a great deal of unification is possible.

[10] See a discussion of the relationship between case studies and theory development pioneered by Alexander George (George and Bennett, 2005) and work urging synthesis of qualitative and quantitative methods (Sambanis, 2004).

macroscopic variables while omitting important detailed variables.[11] In a blistering critique of one version of current methods in the study of intervention operations, social scientist Stathis Kalyvas (Kalyvas, 2008) observed:

> [T]he problems of econometric studies are well known: their main findings are incredibly sensitive to coding and measurement procedures . . . ; they entail a considerable distance between theoretical constructs and proxies . . . as well as multiple observationally equivalent pathways; they suffer from endogeneity . . . ; they lack clear micro foundations or are based on erroneous ones . . . ; and, finally, they are subject to narrow (and untheorized) scope conditions.

### Need to Confront Uncertainty

The need to consider uncertainties is commonly accepted and has long been noted, sometimes with rueful admission that progress in actually doing so has been slow.[12] What it means for models to be able to deal well with uncertainty, however, is not well understood across the scientific community. That said, much progress has been made, and the methods can be brought over into social-behavioral work as discussed in Chapters 5 and 7.

### Subtleties of and Connections Among Model Types

It is generally recognized that *many* types of models will continue to be needed, with diverse attributes.[13] The number of existing types is not

---

[11]  As an example, consider an attempt to find correlates of success (e.g., reducing the number of insurgent attacks) in counterinsurgency operations in Iraq and Afghanistan. If the analysis looks at numbers of intervention forces versus time but ignores the commander's (and insurgent commander's) strategies versus time, correlational results may be meaningless. One way this might happen is if the counterinsurgency commander becomes more aggressive with additional forces, causing more battles to occur, or if increased intervention forces cause the local population to react with alarm toward the invasion by foreigners.

[12]  The 2008 NRC report highlighted uncertainty as an issue. An early reference deploring the tendency of even sharp analysts to deal with uncertainty is a paper by Edward Quade (Quade, 1968) in a book on RAND-style systems analysis (Quade and Boucher, 1968).

[13]  The range of models today is much the same as in the NRC study (Zacharias et al., 2008).

some random development but the result of different contexts and purposes of use. The many attributes usually discussed can be appreciated by asking these questions of models:

- Are they qualitative, semi-qualitative, or quantitative?
- Are they static or dynamic; and, if dynamic, do they use simulation (discrete or continuous) or do they use analytic expressions?
- Are they deterministic or probabilistic?
- What formalism do they use (e.g., influence diagrams, cognitive maps, causal-loop diagrams, factor trees, system dynamics, agent-based modeling, network modeling)?
- At what scales do they apply and—even at given scale—with what degree of abstraction?

What is *not* well understood is how the various model types, formalisms, and scales relate to each other and how they should be used to inform or complement each other. Descriptive comparisons exist, and it is possible to connect many of them in multimodeling,[14] but the underlying phenomenological theory (as distinct from software methods) is not well developed. Challenges are discussed further in Chapter 4, which compares an idealized system view of the real and model worlds and reality versus the ideal.

Some of the questions that arise are: When can models be integrated; when do multimodels make sense; when should one instead use one type of model to generate inputs for another; when are models comparably valid but largely or entirely incommensurate?

### Connecting Theory with Evidence

If theory and both empirical and computational experimentation are the pillars of science, as presented in Figure 1.2, it is hardly controversial to say that they should be well connected. Theory should inform observation, and experimentation should affect theory iteratively and

---

[14] Multimodeling refers to modeling in which a number of models, often expressed in different formalisms, are combined to operate coherently, which requires valid connections among the component models (Levis, 2016). Multimodeling may include integrated human-interface features (Fishwick, 2004).

constructively. However, we believe it evident that scientific and ana-lytic inquiry in the social-behavioral sciences is out of kilter in this respect. The linkages are often not very strong.[15]

Improving the linkages may prove controversial because of deep-seated differences in philosophy between those who are data driven and those who are theory driven. We come back to these matters in Chapters 4 and 5.

### Modularity and Composability

Advances in achieving interoperability among models have been a tri-umph of computer science, significantly due to DARPA investments over decades. Sometimes this is achieved with integrated designs and sometimes with multimodel methods or other devices.[16] In any case, it is now a relatively mature activity.

To achieve *meaningful composition* is a different matter.[17] At a simple level, suppose that model B requires an input X, which model A is said to provide as an output. A and B can then be connected and "run." Suppose, however, that model A's variable X has the same label as the input to B, but is actually quite different (e.g., military force ratio means something quite different to a theater commander than to the officer in charge of a battalion-level engagement). Or suppose that X "means" the same thing, but is measured in different units. Or, more subtle, suppose that model A calculates X using assump-tions that seemed to the model builder reasonable, but were actually valid only for the context of his immediate work, with model B

---

[15] As one example, Steven Zech and Michael Gabbay observed in a paper that "the most striking feature of social network analysis on militants is the lack of overlap between the theoretical and empirical research" (Zech and Gabbay, 2016).

[16] A literature exists on multimodeling and related matters (Fishwick and Zeigler, 1992; Mingers and Gill, 1997; Kött and Citrenbaum, 2010; Tolk, 2012b; Levis, 2016).

[17] An NRC report (National Research Council, 2006) updated initial work (Davis and Anderson, 2003), sharpened issues, and improved the language for discussing different types of difficulty (e.g., syntax, semantics broadly, and pragmatics). Some work dealing with prag-matics occurs within the topic of data engineering (Zeigler and Hammond, 2007). One strand of work has sought to unify the subjects of interoperability and composability by referring to different levels of interoperability (Tolk et al., 2013; Taylor et al., 2015).

requiring an estimate of X that comes from a different concept of how X comes about.[18] In several of the latter cases, A and B can be combined and will run (i.e., they interoperate), but the composition makes no sense.[19] Successful composition depends on the modelers and their understanding of both context and the models to be composed. Obviously, it will be easier to the extent that the separate models are transparent, comprehensible, well documented, and verified. That will be more feasible to the extent that the right methods and technology exist.

Unfortunately, model composition often demands a deeper and more subtle understanding of multiple domains than is realized by those doing the composing. Further, pressures often exist to make the composition happen, to do a quick once-over to establish alleged validity, and to demonstrate its glories. Strong pressures also often exist to standardize as much as possible—i.e., to agree on and hold fixed the values of tuning parameters for both component models and relations among them. All of this is a recipe for failure when attempting to model complex social-behavioral phenomena.[20]

A related issue is that of model federations. We are less sanguine about model federations than was the 2008 NRC report. Indeed, we are somewhat negative rather than merely skeptical. Our views have been influenced by personal experiences and that of colleagues in other organizations. Two problems involve assuring responsibility and the dangers of overstandardization as discussed in what follows.

---

[18] Examples of potentially hidden assumptions include rational-analytic decisionmaking, system equilibrium in economics, or a flat-earth approximation.

[19] See discussions in the literature (Tolk, 2012b; Yilmaz and Ören, 2006; Yilmaz, 2006b; Yilmaz et al., 2007; and Yilmaz and Ören, 2009).

[20] We thank Cory Lofdahl for related discussions (see also Lofdahl, 2010). The problems of dealing with a multiplicity of "tuning parameters" are hardly unique to social-behavioral modeling. They arise, for example, in the modeling of climate change. See Koonin, 2014, and the heated debate about the controversial article (most easily found by web browsing). The continuing dispute may lead to a "Red Team/Blue Team" review organized by the Environmental Protection Agency (Plumer and Davenport, 2017).

### Good Analysis Requires Taking Responsibility

In our experience, analytic studies that attempt to give good information and sometimes advice to senior leaders require tight control of all the analytic components by the analytic team. They must thoroughly understand the models, data, uncertainties, and implications of model outputs. They are *responsible* for doing so. This is altogether different from "demonstrating" a method that combines multiple models and data sources. It has certainly proved valuable to compose models in a group's local federation, but doing so in a meaningful way has required substantial effort to understand subtleties, make code-level adjustments, and ensure validity for the narrow purpose of the study, which in turn requires continuity of key personnel and tight working relationships.[21] In contrast, we have observed demonstrations of alleged analytic capability in which—despite heroic efforts by those involved—the resulting program was at best good enough for the particular details of the demonstration case and fragile otherwise. We are especially leery of large multiparty confederations if results are to be used analytically because such confederations inevitably spread responsibility.

A counterargument is the claim that some of today's problems are too complicated for any one mind to fathom, or even one small team. Multidisciplinary efforts are necessary, along with trust. Multimodeling and federations then follow naturally. We remain skeptical—especially given difficulties when working relationships are constrained by parties protecting intellectual property (e.g., by proving black-box component models with encrypted "innards") or when time is short.

### The Dangers of Over-Standardization

We have also been influenced by the negative effects of DoD having become dependent on large, complicated, and standardized "campaign models" of warfare. In 2011, the DoD disestablished a large group responsible for such modeling and analysis. As discussed in a congressionally mandated review, the monolithic, highly standardized approach had proved to be a recipe for overly narrow, incomprehensible,

---

[21] For examples, see Matsumura et al., 2001; Steeb et al., 2011; and a discussion of the COMPOEX program (Kött and Citrenbaum, 2010).

uncertain *insensitive* analysis serving policymakers poorly (P. Davis, 2016). The models themselves were not the culprit and they could in fact be understood by specialists, but the inexorable effect of standardization is often to suppress uncertainty, even when dealing with uncertainty is crucial to analysis.

To summarize, with some repetition, it is necessary to better understand how to achieve *meaningful* model compositions, but the goal should not be "blessed federations" and databases, but the ability to compose models appropriately for a given purpose and context, while allowing for uncertainty, disagreement, and competition. That is, a composition should be "fit for purpose." This should be much easier with community-available libraries with well-vetted modules (including competitive modules) available for various aspects of social-behavioral theory. A major issue is what those modules should be and how they should be developed, peer-reviewed, and shared.[22] Two general admonitions apply:

- No general solution exists for ensuring that a composition is meaningful. This situation will not change with a new technology.
- It is more reasonable to educate modelers and analysts about subtleties and then to seek relatively general *processes and procedures* by which to validate a composition for a given context and to identify methods and tools to help. That is, it is more reasonable to seek processes and procedures to assess "fitness for purpose."

## Rethinking Model Validity
### The Five Dimensions of Model Validity
Given the difficulties in measuring faithfully the many variables important to human and social behavior, and given the difficulty and sometimes

---

[22] One study illustrated an unusual approach. It began with a factor-tree qualitative model based on a review of social science literature on public support for terrorism. It then mapped the factor tree into a semi-qualitative computational model to use for exploration. This required specifying numerous alternative algorithms and other subtleties. This was accomplished with a very high-level language, with the expectation that this social science module could be peer-reviewed without the diversions of computer-code details. If the model proved solid, it could be readily shared, used for multimodeling purposes, or reprogrammed into languages more convenient to particular groups (Davis and O'Mahony, 2013).

the impossibility of predicting CAS behavior, it is necessary to redefine "validity" of theories and models. Much discussion has already occurred (see Appendix C), and it is time to draw conclusions and move on rather than debate the matters endlessly. Fortunately, it is possible to proceed by merely extending the classic concept.

Official definitions are often disappointing, but the DoD's definition of validation (Department of Defense, 2009) has held up for decades:

> Validation: The process of determining the degree to which a model and its associated data are an accurate representation of the real world from the perspective of the intended uses of the model.[23]

We propose the following *elaboration*: A model's validity should be assessed separately with respect to (1) description, (2) causal explanation, (3) postdiction, (4) exploratory analysis, and (5) prediction.

These criteria should be elaborated and better defined in future work, but we have the following meanings in mind:

- Description: identify salient structure, variables, and processes.
- Causal explanation: identify causal variables and processes and describe reasons for behavior in corresponding terms.
- Postdiction: explain past behavior quantitatively with inferences from causal theory.
- Exploratory analysis: identify and parameterize causal variables and processes. Estimate approximate system behavior as a function of those parameters and variations of model structure (coarse prediction).
- Prediction: predict system behavior accurately and even precisely (as assessed with empirical information).

We need not elaborate on description or prediction, but the other dimensions bear somewhat more commentary. Causal explanation is at once a familiar and primitive concept, but is also deep and subtle as is

---

[23] This DoD definition is consistent with most other thoughtful discussions, such as that in the domain of system dynamics (Sterman, 2000).

discussed in Chapter 5 in the section on causality. Let us elaborate here on postdiction and exploratory analysis.

*Postdiction* (sometimes called "retrodiction") can have the negative connotation of after-the-fact rationalization, but we have in mind the positive connotation of explaining previously observed system behavior using theory. Physicist Steven Weinberg uses the example of Einstein's explanation of the observed anomaly in Mercury's orbit. Weinberg describes that as more important and persuasive in science than subsequent predictions (Weinberg, 1994, p. 96ff.). Explaining Mercury's behavior was in part persuasive to physicists because of the theory's elegance.[24] Persuasion occurred even though agreement of Einstein's predictions with subsequent empirical data was equivocal for years. Geological science, of course, also depends on postdiction. A more recent example might be that economists can persuasively explain the economic crash of 2007–2008 by looking at information about the state of the economy and central bank policies before the crash—information that was available in principle beforehand, but that was not adequately appreciated at the time.[25] In retrospect, the crash was avoidable (Financial Crisis Inquiry Commission, 2011).

*Exploratory analysis* and coarse prediction refer to studying the model's behavior over the uncertain space of inputs (also called scenario space),[26] perhaps to identify regions with "good" and "bad" characteristics.

---

[24] A pure expression of this comes from the great physicist Paul Adrien Maurice Dirac, who wrote: "The physicist, in his study of natural phenomena, has two methods of making progress: (1) the method of experiment and observation, and (2) the method of mathematical reasoning. . . . There is no logical reason why the second method should be possible at all, but one has found in practice that it does work and meets with reasonable success. This must be ascribed to some mathematical quality of Nature, a quality which the casual observer of Nature would not expect, but which nevertheless plays an important role in Nature's scheme" (Dirac, 1939). Dirac went on to emphasize the importance of mathematical beauty, something he regards as no more definable than beauty in art, but something that people who study mathematics have no difficulty in appreciating. How well this applies to social science remains to be seen.

[25] Some individuals were exceptions, saw the signals, and profited handsomely, as recounted in the book and movie *The Big Short* (Lewis, 2010).

[26] The related concepts of exploratory analysis and exploratory modeling (Davis and Finch, 1993; Bankes, 1993; Davis, 1994) are core elements of analysis addressing "deep uncertainty," as discussed later in this report. As increasingly emphasized in recent work, exploratory

The purpose is not to *predict* what will happen, but to understand what *may* happen and to estimate the circumstances under which various behaviors are most likely. But how might one judge validity for such purposes? An early suggestion stated:

> A model and its case space (databases) is valid for exploratory analysis if the case space represents well the degree of uncertainty in inputs and, within that case space, the model is either structurally valid, behaves in ways adequately consistent with what is known empirically, or is based on what appear to be reasonable assumptions. As always in a discussion of validity adequacy must be judged in the context of the particular application. (Bigelow and Davis, 2003, p. 19)

An example of "coarse prediction" might be using a model to identify high-risk regions of a system's state space, without purporting to predict precisely what the system would do in that region. For a social phenomenon, that characterization of state might involve, for example, the fraction of the population with a particular attitude or behavior, the efficiency of communications within the population, and the existence of "sparks."

Figure 2.1 illustrates how a model might be characterized in this five-dimensional framework. The notional model is said to be descriptive, to have a good sense of the causal variables and processes, to be good for postdiction and exploratory analysis, but to be poor for prediction. Why the latter? Perhaps the values of the key causal variables are not known currently—i.e., they are knowable in principle at some point, but are uncertain currently. This circumstance is common in strategic planning and in social science. It is the reason that so much social science is expressed in contingent terms. That "wishy-washiness" may make decisionmakers unhappy, but predicting the details of future states of the world is often not in the cards. In such cases, "good" theory is contingent, not narrowly predictive.

---

analysis needs to consider uncertainties in the model itself—i.e., structural uncertainties (Davis et al., 2016)—not just the parameter values of a given model.

**Figure 2.1**
**Spider Chart Characterization of a Model's Validity by Five Criteria**

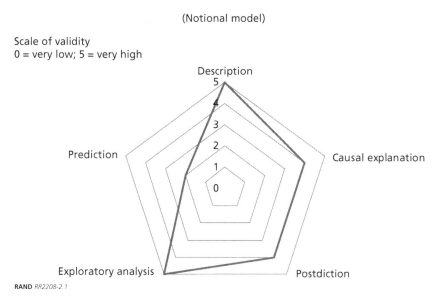

RAND RR2208-2.1

Other models would have very different spider-diagram characteristics. For example, some models are predictive but not descriptive with respect to causal variables (as when epidemiological models use proxies such as temperature and humidity rather than mosquito populations or when macroeconomic models predicting next year's rise in gross domestic product have no obvious relationship to underlying microeconomic mechanisms).

### Assessing a Model's Validity in a Context

As has long been understood, validity can only be judged for a purpose and context: What is being asked of the model and what are the circumstances? For example, is the model being asked whether a policy intervention will have a positive effect or what the magnitude of that effect will be? Is the question being asked when the state of the system is near equilibrium and the intervention effects would be marginal and captured by elasticities, or is it being asked when the system is "on the edge of chaos"?

A related question is whether the system in question has "stationary behavior" or whether its structure or basic relationships are changing. Weather models were long considered to be statistically valid, as in characterizing once-in-a-century storms. They are no longer valid because the frequency of high-intensity storms is increasing, presumably due to climate change.[27] As a second example, classic two-party American political models are no longer valid because so many individuals regard themselves as independent. Further, polarization has increased with the disappearance of "moderates."[28]

### Notional Comparison of Models

Figure 2.2 shows a notional depiction of how some models might be characterized using the framework of Figure 2.1. It adds a distinction between systems that are stable and systems that are changing (right and left sides, respectively, in Figure 2.2). The numbers are notional, but the intent is to convey the idea that classic equilibrium theory in economics is good when used to deal with a stable world (right side). So also, empirical models, such as from machine intelligence or econometrics, can be very predictive in such circumstances, but be poor in terms of providing causal explanation. Looking to the left side of Figure 2.2, both classes of model are poor when the world is changing in fundamental ways.[29] An agent-based model might do better by having adaptive agents representing causes of major change (e.g., societal changes of taste, sentiment, or even basic values), but would be afflicted by so many parametric uncertainties as to make prediction rough at best. A hybrid model (If only we knew how to build it) might have the best features of both.

---

[27] Fortunately, weather forecasters understand this because they routinely get empirical feedback about their predictions. Thus, they enjoy a quick, tight, repeated cycle.

[28] See polling results by the Pew Research Center. See, e.g., its report from June 12, 2014, "Political Polarization in the American Public."

[29] A related concept is whether a system's processes can be regarded as "stationary." This terminology has a variety of meanings depending on discipline. In statistics, a system is stationary if its relevant joint probability distributions are constant. In decision analysis, an issue is whether the actors' utility functions (if they exist at all) are constant.

**Figure 2.2**
**Notional Comparison of Model Validities**

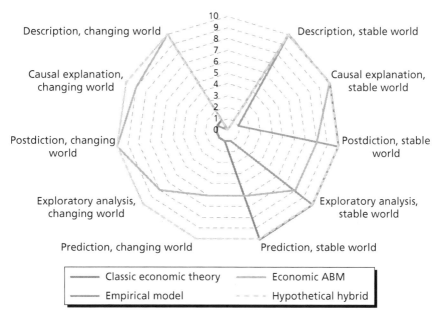

NOTE: This variant of a spider or radar diagram juxtaposes (left to right) notional dimensions of a
model's validity for stable-world and changing-world results. To accomplish this, the topmost
vertex is left blank.
RAND RR2208-2.2

Discussions of validity, then, can be richer in the multidimensional
approach. Far more work is needed to turn the vision into a methodology. As of today, no agreement exists on the details of Figures 2.1 or
2.2—i.e., on how to define the individual dimensions for quantitative or qualitative measurement or how adequately to specify context,
including what decision is to be aided (Chapter 7).

### Differences Between the Physical and Social Sciences

By using the five dimensions of validity we may also see that the difference between validating models for the physical and social sciences is
often not as great as usually claimed. For example, the "fundamental
laws of physics" are seldom predictively valid for real-world applications. Rather, as discussed by Nancy Cartwright, they are remarkably
descriptive and explanatory about idealized systems. When employed

for real-world purposes, they are typically modified and adjusted because the real world departs from the ideal (Cartwright, 1983). That is, context matters greatly, as it does in the social sciences.

### Some General Criteria for Validation

Theorists and modelers have been struggling with the issue of validation for many years. A good deal of de facto consensus exists at the practical level. Some methods apply to each of the five dimensions discussed above. Our summary is that we make judgments (whether of theories or models) about validity or what might better be called confidence based on the following:[30]

1. Falsifiability (if a mode cannot be falsified, it fails as meaningful science).
2. Roots in deeper theory regarded as valid.
3. Logic (e.g., does the model have internal validity?).
4. Confirmational evidence, especially model successes in cases chosen to attempt falsification, but in broad patterns of success.
5. Elegance and logic. Theoretical physicists are famous or notorious for their attention to matters such as coherence and beauty. Others look for consistency and power of description and explanation.
6. Due diligence. Since judgment is involved, a key is whether we applied due diligence in considering all of the foregoing.

We end this discussion of validation with some admonitions for sponsors and managers of model-building research. First, we note that the issue is, essentially, a matter of quality assurance. A strong lesson from other disciplines is that the prime determinant of quality at the end is quality along the way, which is the result of top-notch people and good organizational environments. A principle that is generally helpful is to require clean conceptual models early for peer review, debate,

---

[30] How these criteria fit together, and the limitations of each, is discussed by philosopher Susan Haack (Haack, 2011). She skewers those "New Cynics" who erroneously go from true statements such as "Theories are not implied by their positive instances" to what amounts to "All theories are equal" (see pp. 34–35).

and iteration (see also Chapter 4, "Reality versus the Ideal"). Representing the resulting model in a comprehensible language is desirable and, in any case, should be accomplished with best practices (e.g., structuring, documentation, and routine verification). Lastly, we note that organizations may seek to validate models for whole classes of application, which is problematic because validity must be judged by details of how it is to be used (e.g., is the model valid for establishing whether option A or option B is superior, in a set of test cases, as characterized by particular measures of effectiveness?). Thus, establishing validity is not something for specialists; rather, it a core part of the responsibility of analysts using models to inform decisions.

# CHAPTER THREE

# Broad Strategy for Next Steps

To address the problems of earlier sections, we recommend that DARPA should define two or three difficult national challenge problems for multi-year efforts forcing productive inter- and trans-disciplinary work in useful directions.

The motivation would be as for other historical "grand challenges." Examples in mathematics go back to Euclid and include David Hilbert's twenty-three problems expressed in 1900. Hilbert asked:

> Who among us would not be glad to lift the veil behind which the future lies hidden; to cast a glance at the next advances of our science and at the secrets of its development during future centuries? (Carlson et al., 2006, p. 22)

Grand challenges help focus minds and energize. Their concreteness is part of their allure. We see such challenges as important for DARPA's pursuits in social-behavioral research because the subject area is so broad and shapeless: some temporary narrowing could be helpful if meeting the challenges would "lift the veil" on important matters. How to choose the right grand challenges is a matter for subsequent discussion, but some possibilities with national importance include understanding and finding ways to counter:

- Radicalization for terrorism
- Weakening of democracy and national cohesion by foreign information operations campaigns
- Prospects for stability after international interventions

- Behaviors of populations after natural disasters
- Opioid or obesity epidemics

The gamut ranges from national security topics to those of a broader and more social-policy character. A principle should be defining problems in such a way as to breed a dynamic, creative, cross-pollinating, knowledge-building culture.

For *each* such national challenge, DARPA would post concrete challenges in five subcategories.[1]

1. Challenge social-behavioral scientists to generate more unifying and coherent theories while retaining and sharpening alternative perspectives.
2. Ensure that models represent the best theories faithfully, which includes addressing shortcomings of past modeling repeatedly pointed out by social scientists. This will often require tending to context-specific aspects of phenomena and recognizing stochastic factors.
3. Challenge experimenters to find new theory-informed ways to obtain relevant information and analyze the data—*coordinating* empirical and computational experimentation in a way that reflects their comparative strengths and weaknesses and exploits new empirical sources.
4. Challenge other theorists and technologists to provide new methods and tools to improve capabilities for the above subcategories, including comprehensible visualizations of systems and their behavior characteristics across the n-dimensional system state space, and to tailor them to the needs of analysis in application work.
5. Improve and nurture the rest of the ecology needed for overall effectiveness (i.e., infrastructure, culture, and governance).

Figure 3.1 reminds us that the challenges apply to all the activities within the ecology. Even though most researchers will be fully occu-

---

[1] This approach is different from that in more typical DARPA challenge problems (e.g., get an autonomous vehicle to drive a specified distance on a specified road network).

**Figure 3.1**
**The Ecology to Respond to National Challenges**

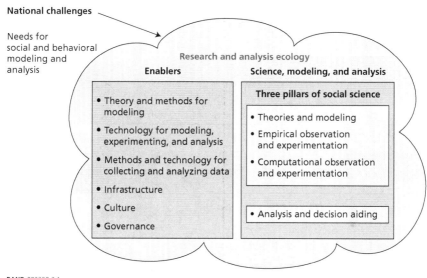

National challenges

Needs for social and behavioral modeling and analysis

Research and analysis ecology

**Enablers**

- Theory and methods for modeling
- Technology for modeling, experimenting, and analysis
- Methods and technology for collecting and analyzing data
- Infrastructure
- Culture
- Governance

**Science, modeling, and analysis**

**Three pillars of social science**

- Theories and modeling
- Empirical observation and experimentation
- Computational observation and experimentation

- Analysis and decision aiding

RAND *RR2208-3.1*

pied within their part(s) of the ecology, DARPA will need to be concerned about the totality to have a more holistic view.

For each such national challenge taken on, it might be useful to construct a kind of virtual social-behavioral modeling laboratory (SBML), somewhat analogous to the creation of task forces.[2] Figure 3.2 suggests the basic idea; the concept is discussed at more length in Appendix A. Briefly, such a "laboratory" would exist for a finite time (e.g., five to ten years), during which it would strive for a maximum degree

---

[2] In contemplating an SBML, we can learn much from transformation efforts in business. These efforts sometimes address many generic issues raised in this report, such as (1) working with stakeholders to understand their concerns; (2) identifying the key physical and social phenomena across multiple scales; (3) developing systemic conceptual models (often qualitative visualizations) to understand key relationships and discuss with stakeholders; (4) parametric modeling; (5) testing; and (6) application. See particularly a review by William Rouse (Rouse, 2015) relating to health care systems.

of sharing and synergism in interdisciplinary activities.[3] Some features are important to highlight. First, this approach would be dynamic and iterative, with routine competition and iteration and with multiple strands of work. It would *not* be an attempt to construct a single, monolithic federation of the allegedly correct models with the allegedly correct data. Models would be composed as appropriate for research and analysis purposes. Any such compositions would need to be validated accordingly as "fit for purpose." Second, we envision numerous kinds of models, including simulation, but also human gaming, analytic modeling, and other varieties. Some of the modeling would be qualitative, some would be quantitative. Conference discussions would be very much about the national challenge, related social science, the degree to which modeling represents that science, the quality of data from both empirical and computational experimentation, and how to characterize knowledge to inform decisions about the particular grand challenge (e.g., whether a particular intervention would reduce the number of jihadi recruits or whether certain doctrinal procedures in disaster relief would help or hurt).[4] Again, then, a challenge problem would force boundary-crossing, communication, and synthesis.

Another important aspect of the boundary-crossing is getting out of the laboratory (or office) to become thoroughly familiar with problems "on the ground" and concerns of the various stakeholders that would be affected by any interventions. One of the great strengths of a problem-focused approach is that it encourages this practice. Some of its manifestations may include participative modeling and changes in the variables considered by both theory-oriented and experiment-oriented researchers and analysts.[5]

---

[3]  The concept could be described simply as an unusually coherent program, but the term "laboratory" conveys the sense of purposeful experimentation on a particular problem.

[4]  Empirically, American jihadists have diverse backgrounds as discussed in a paper by Brian Jenkins (Jenkins, 2017). Such data should inform judgments about intervention.

[5]  Some related literature includes an influential book by Bent Flyvbjerg (Flyvbjerg, 2001) and related debate (Flyvbjerg, 2004; Laitin, 2003) and a "practical" book by Richard Swedberg (Swedberg, 2014). The system dynamics literature emphasizes close interaction with stakeholders (Sterman, 2000), and the subject of "collaborative modeling" has become a topic in sustainability research and related areas (Olabisi et al., 2015). Stakeholder engage-

**Figure 3.2**
**An SBML for a Particular National Challenge**

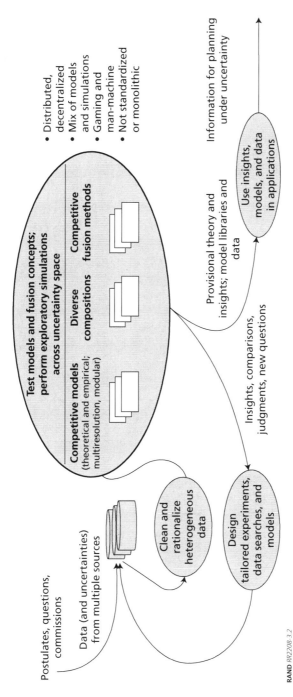

RAND RR2208-3.2

A successful SBML approach would foster a new "epistemic culture" (arrangements and mechanisms by which we gain knowledge) in social-behavioral research: Those participating would be building knowledge in a very different and more multifaceted way than is customary within discipline-bound inquiry. The result would reflect not just scientific knowledge and craft, but also what Aristotle called *phronesis* (virtuous thoughtful and practical doing that reflects an understanding of ethics and situational subtleties). We see such practical doing as including the confrontation of uncertainty and expecting to adapt as necessary. The word may be Greek, but the ideas endure.[6]

This concludes our discussion of general approach. Subsequent chapters go deeper. First, Chapter 4 discusses broadly how to improve linkages among theory, modeling, and experimentation in the course of the research cycle. Chapters 5–9 discuss more discrete challenges for science, modeling, decision aiding, methods, culture, and infrastructure.

---

ment was a core element in RAND work that supported the development and passage of a master plan for Louisiana's post-Katrina efforts (Fischbach, 2010; Groves et al., 2013) and in numerous efforts to improve the health care system (Rouse, 2015).

[6] The value of phronesis is argued in the philosophical literature by policy practitioners such as Bent Flyvbjerg (Flyvbjerg and Landman, 2012). How scientific cultures can be quite distinct is illustrated by an ethnographic comparison of high-energy physics and molecular biology (Knorr-Cetina, 1999). Some of the most interesting portions of the book are endnotes with post-text dialogue between the author and scientists with whom the author had communicated during her initial research (e.g., pp. 270–290). A vibrant version of the SBML approach would encourage what professor of informatics Bonne Nardi discusses under the rubrics of activity theory and distributed cognition (Nardi, 1996).

# CHAPTER FOUR

# Tightening the Theory-Modeling-Experimentation Research Cycle

A significant obstacle in pursuing the objectives discussed in this report is improving linkages among the three pillars shown in Figure 1.2. Before describing our suggestions, it is useful to provide background to help explain the current state of affairs. This requires a digression into the philosophy of science, even though it is doubtful that said philosophy helps scientists do their work.[1]

## Background on Differences of Philosophy

Although researchers are usually too busy to be waxing philosophical, two reasonably distinct tribes can be observed. The tribes differ in their thinking about the nature of science, the scientific method, and the meaning of truth. They also use different methods and have different conceptions of what constitutes good and bad method. Their incentive structures may be more about in-discipline activity than problem solving. Understanding all this will be an important part of moving forward expeditiously with the kinds of national challenge discussed earlier. As one of our team members (Gulden) noted ruefully from his own experience, interdisciplinary work

---

[1]  Nobelist and physicist Steven Weinberg writes about this in a chapter entitled "Against Philosophy" (Weinberg, 1994). He approves of philosopher Ludwig Wittgenstein, who remarked that "nothing seems to me less likely than that a scientist or mathematician who reads me should be seriously influenced in the way he works" (Weinberg, p. 167). Weinberg doth protest too much, since the reader will find that he has obviously spent a great deal of time reading philosophy.

in academia can take a very long time: Months and numerous meetings may occur before, eventually, participants understand where others are coming from and how to communicate. With this in mind, some digression into philosophy of science is worthwhile.

The related literature in question is rich, provocative, and enjoyable to review from time to time (not as a steady diet). One important conclusion is that *the notion of "scientific method" is a myth.* In his seminal book on inquiry for the social sciences, Abraham Kaplan quipped:

> This book will contain no definition of "scientific method." . . . There is no one thing to be defined . . . one could as well speak of "the method" for baseball. (Kaplan, 1964, p. 27)

Scientific method is ultimately a *body* of techniques for investigating phenomena. Application of the techniques is anything but simple, linear, and formulaic. Variations of style are notable. Similarly, how science progresses, and how the ideas and theories emerge, is often complex and erratic, which is a theme of Thomas Kuhn (Kuhn, 1970) and the philosophical bomb thrower Paul Feyerabend, whose book, entitled *Against Method*, is sometimes paraphrased as "Anything goes!" (Feyerabend, 1975).

Susan Haack expresses similar disdain for the notion of scientific method, arguing that the methods of science can be seen as critical common sense (Haack, 2011). That is, the methods are like those we apply routinely but—crucially—are "conducted with greater care, detail, precision, and persistence" (p. 7). She mentions similar views of Albert Einstein and Thomas Huxley and notes that she sees science as very much like working crossword puzzles (as did Einstein). She also notes the fundamental importance of integrity in scientific research.[2]

Fortunately, consensus exists on some principles if inquiry is to be regarded as scientific. The principles relate to reproducibility, falsifiability, and adherence to certain principles of reasoning. Again, the principles

---

[2]   Many readers will have studied the ideas of Karl Popper, Imre Lakatos, and perhaps Paul Feyerabend in college. If so, we recommend Susan Haack's work as a critical review and synthesis with important additions. Along the way, she points out bitingly but humorously contradictions in the thinking of the earlier philosophers and how they evolved (Haack, 2011).

**Table 4.1**
**Two Views About Fundamentals**

| View One (Scientific Realism) | View Two (Constructivism) |
| --- | --- |
| Reality exists and science seeks to understand it. | Reality is socially constructed and relative. |
| Empirical data tells us about reality. | Empirical data is meaningful only through one or another interpretation. Interpretations vary markedly. |
| Theories build and expand on each other. | Theories supplant each other over time (often when adherents of earlier theory die off). |
| With effort, relatively general theory should emerge, creating increased coherence. | Theories are and will continue to be incommensurate, exquisitely contextual, and resistant to generalization. |
| Science converges toward truth. | Science evolves erratically and should not be assumed to be converging on anything, much less truth. |

are not unique to science, but they are more assiduously followed in science.

Despite these points of consensus, it is useful to discern two camps. Dichotomous discussion is always dangerous, but it highlights differences due to backgrounds, assumptions, languages, and intuitions. Even within our author team we saw the dichotomy, as our academic backgrounds include theoretical chemistry and physics, engineering, political science and economics, policy analysis, and anthropology. Table 4.1 contrasts the two views, sometimes referred to in shorthand as *scientific realism* and *constructivism*.[3] By and large, physical scientists and engineers lean more toward View One and social scientists lean more toward View Two.

The dichotomy has implications for social-behavioral modeling. The constructivist view would seem to be potentially hostile to the notion that modeling even makes sense. At a minimum, those in its tribe tend to be skeptical (often for good reason) about modeling and

---

[3]   See a short article on "Scientific Objectivity" in *The Stanford Encyclopedia* (Reiss and Sprinter, 2017).

(as noted in Table 4.1) even the notion of progress in science.[4] The scientific-realism view, in its extreme, can be dogmatic. For example, classic economic theory exalts the notion of the rational actor maximizing subjective expected utility and also the notion that all values can be monetized to permit such an optimization. Anthropologists, sociologists, and social psychologists are likely to cringe at such notions.[5]

Table 4.2 explains the tack we take. The first column reflects a naysayer view; the second column describes our approach, which we see as pragmatic. It preemptively accepts that it would be folly to imagine that good social-behavioral modeling can be like normal engineering, that it will lend itself to traditional prediction, that there is only one good way to look at a social system, or that we should anticipate achieving the kind of control over the system that is possible when dealing with the objects of standard engineering.

This operational approach looks like scientific realism, which provides frameworks for framing issues and moving forward. However, if pursued properly it will address practical and legitimate concerns associated with constructivism. This may not satisfy inveterate constructivists, but we hope that it provides a middle ground in which they will at least be willing to operate provisionally.

The tack suggested has precedent. The field of system dynamics has dealt with soft variables for more than a half century.[6] Also, what we regard as good policy analysis emphasizes that good analysis must recognize and honor alternative value frames. Good policy analysis frames the issues so that the varied considerations are *all* visible and evaluates options accordingly. The decisions themselves reflect the criteria that people choose to emphasize and judgments that those people make.[7]

---

[4]   Debates on such matters have been strong within academic anthropology, as discussed by Lawrence Kuznar in a book critical of postmodernist thinking and its sometimes-paralyzing effects on the field (Kuznar, 2008).

[5]   So also, modern financial experts such as Richard Bookstaber have moved far beyond classic economics in their thinking (Bookstaber, 2017).

[6]   See Forrester (1963) or a comprehensive textbook (Sterman, 2000).

[7]   Full objectivity is an aspiration, but a hallmark of science is vigorous pursuit of that aspiration (Haack, 2011, p. 25).

**Table 4.2**
**Proposed Tack**

| Initial View | Pragmatism |
|---|---|
| 1. Progress is an illusion. | Let's work with the illusion. |
| 2. Everything is contextual, so theory is doubtful. | Absolutely, but what are the variables that define context? How far can we go in identifying and in some cases measuring them, even if roughly? |
| 3. Truth is an illusion. Many truths exist. | Let us assume that truth is multifaceted and appears very different through alternative lenses. Some lenses reflect different values. But how far can we go in revealing and relating those different facets and perspectives? Should we not be able to describe and work with all of them? |
| 4. Theories are incommensurate and equally "valid" in their own way. | Let's see what theories can be reconciled, combined, or related. Perhaps some will indeed remain incommensurate. But let's see. Some theories will be falsifiable. |
| 5. Social systems are chaotic complex adaptive systems; they are chaotic and not subject to prediction. | A complex adaptive system is not always chaotic; its state may variously be relatively stable, potentially unstable, or highly unstable to interventions or other new events. Even in unstable states, its evolution may be constrained to one of some trajectories that can be anticipated. We do not see "prediction" as an appropriate term, but we can often anticipate possibilities, ascribe some degree of relative likelihood, and/or enjoy *some* degree of control. When? |
| 6. Systems thinking is for engineers; it does not work well for social systems in which context dominates. | Humility is necessary. Drawing the system's boundaries widely may be essential, by including variables and processes that are qualitative or otherwise soft. The purpose of a system model is often more explanatory or exploratory than predictive.[a] |
| 7. Uncertainties are overwhelming. | Much progress has been made in dealing with deep uncertainty. Let's see how far we can get, encouraging major ambitions but maintaining humility (see Chapter 5, "Dealing Routinely with Uncertainty"). |

[a] Lest this be regarded as a defect, we note that Darwin's theory of evolution by natural selection, one of the most profound of scientific contributions, had little predictive to offer.

The next section proceeds in this spirit. It takes a "system view," but not the simple-minded system view that can often be found in modeling that purports to address social-behavioral matters but is actually far too mechanistic.

## An Idealized System View Relating the Real and Model Worlds

Closing the theory-modeling-experimentation gap requires improving interactions among social-behavioral scientists on the one hand and modelers on the other. The problem is implied by the form of the previous sentence, which distinguishes between scientists and modelers. Why are they separate, whereas in other fields they are not? A related challenge is improving the degree to which theories and models can be comprehended, reproduced, debated, and iterated. With these troublesome challenges in mind, we offer an idealized vision to better characterize what we would *like*, so that we can better discuss next steps.

With this background Figure 4.1 depicts a view of the research cycle that is useful for our context. Although significantly adapted here, it draws on prior depictions over the decades, especially by Robert Sargent, Bernard Ziegler, and Andreas Tolk.[8]

Again, Figure 4.1 denotes an *idealized* way of relating the real and model worlds. It comes from a scientific realism perspective but can address many constructivist ideas. *It anticipates that knowledge building will involve a combination of induction, deduction, and abduction.*[9] The imagery is that a real system exists, which is the social system of interest (item 1). Real-world observation and experimentation (item 2) help us in abstracting and in forming hypotheses about the system's elements, relationships, and processes. Because theory and modeling are always

---

[8]   Distinctions between conceptual model and implementation are discussed in early papers and texts (Sargent, 2010; Zeigler et al., 2000; Sargent, 1984; Zeigler, 1984). Zeigler also introduced the crucial concept of "experimental frame," specifying conditions under which the real and model systems are to be observed and how model results are to be used. More recent work has sharpened relationships between system engineering and modeling theory (Tolk, 2012a), as well as highlighting a difference between a conceptual model and fully specified model (a distinction that many authors choose not to recognize).

[9]   Deduction is deriving a conclusion by reasoning from premises (e.g., from an accepted model); induction is inferring a conclusion by generalizing from particular instances (e.g., as in observing experimental results that suggest patterns); abduction is inference in which subjectively *probable* conclusions are drawn from a mixture of premises, observations, and more uncertain assumptions. Only exceptional models are sound enough to justify depending on deduction, but many models are good enough to support "reasonable" abduction. The concept of abduction was introduced by Charles Sanders Peirce around 1865 (Peirce and Buchler, 1940).

**Figure 4.1**
**An Idealized System View of the Real and Modeled Worlds**

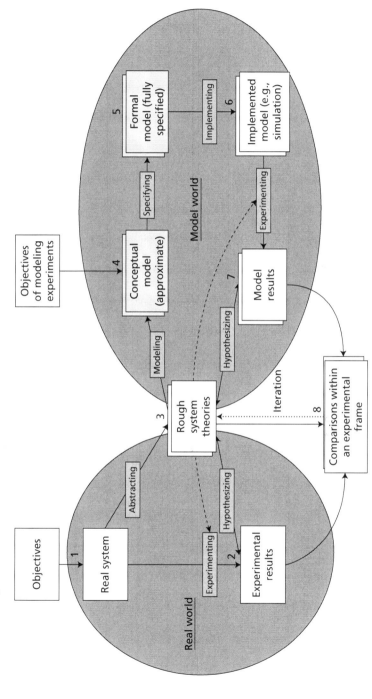

NOTE: Currently, the yellow items (conceptual and formal models) seldom exist separately.

RAND *RR2208-4.1*

simplifications, we must have particular objectives in mind when asking about the real world or how to model it. We then construct rough-cut system theories in our heads to approximate the relevant reality (item 3). Often, alternative notions about the system exist, reflecting different hypotheses, perspectives, or both. This is symbolized in Figure 4.1 by the stacking of icons.

Moving rightward, we then construct *coherent* conceptual models (plural) of the system (item 4)—including aspects that are important but cannot be easily observed directly. The conceptual models may be combinations of essays, listings of objects and attributes, or such devices as influence, stock-and-flow, or network diagrams. The next step, which is not always feasible or desirable, is to develop a formal model (item 5)— i.e., one that specifies all the information needed for computation of model consequences, generating consequences for different cases by using lookup tables. That is, a specified model must have tight definitions, equations, algorithms, or tables, as needed.

In this idealized image rooted in classic pedagogy, the formal model is independent of programming language or—far more plausible— expressed in a very high-level language that is easily comprehended by nonprogrammers (i.e., in a week rather than a month). Why? The reason is to lay bare the essence of the model without the mind-muddling complications of most computer code and to permit replication, peer review, debate, and iteration. *After* those occur, a formal model can (moving downward) be implemented in other programming languages as convenient (item 6).[10] Moving leftward, the implemented model can then be used with an experimental design to generate model results across the n-dimensional space of model inputs. Results of these computational experiments (exploratory analysis) may (item 7) falsify or add credence to earlier beliefs and suggest further hypotheses to enrich system theories. For example, they may suggest that the system will show extremely bad behavior in certain circumstances not previously considered

---

[10] Recent literature documents failures to replicate peer-reviewed scientific work (Open Science Collaboration, 2015). Although some authors claim that such accounts have been exaggerated (Gilbert et al., 2016), surveys indicate considerable concern among scientists themselves about replicability.

(i.e., "if more than roughly 10 percent of the social group . . . and . . . occurs . . . then very bad things are likely to happen"). Such important computational conclusions should be compared to experimental results from the real system, shown at the bottom of Figure 4.1 (item 8). To do so sensibly requires defining the relevant experimental frame as defined earlier—i.e., specifying the conditions under which the real and model systems are to be observed and how model results are to be used.[11] A model can be considered valid for a particular application in a particular context if the result of using the model's outputs are adequately close to the result of using the real system's behavior for that experimental frame. Or, more precisely, we consider the model valid if, after due diligence in considering available knowledge,[12] we believe that the model's outputs are adequately close to that of the real system. The cycle continues. Overall, Figure 4.1 conveys a sense of a virtuous research cycle in which theory, model, and implemented model (program) are updated.

Figure 4.1 adapts from earlier work[13] but differs from earlier depictions in some respects:

- It is oriented more to science than engineering: "Objectives" matter in developing and evaluating models within science, but the word "requirements" does not appear because research objectives are often fuzzy as in "understand what is going on. . . ."
- It allows for diverse types of models, not just simulations. For example, it allows for an economist's model predicting steady-state outcomes. The conceptual model may even be qualitative or even graphic.
- It shows theories at pivot points affecting empirical experimentation, computational experimentation, and comparisons. The theories inform what experiments should be conducted and how results should be analyzed.

---

[11] The term "experimental frame" was introduced by Bernard Zeigler in a 1984 textbook on modeling theory, a second edition of which is now available (Zeigler et al., 2000).

[12] See Tolk et al. (2013), where these matters are discussed and related to the theory of language.

[13] The figure benefited from a paper by and discussion with Andreas Tolk (Tolk, 2012b).

- It refers to plural theories because more than one may exist—even more than one intendedly comprehensive theory reflecting different narratives. This is crucial if we are to reflect the markedly different views of reality suggested by, say, anthropologists, economists, or physicists.[14] Sometimes, it means accounting for emotions, history, and sacred values.[15]
- It takes seriously the separate existence of a fully specified model that is either language independent or in a very high-level language comprehensible to social scientists and their graduate students without being serious programmers. This is analogous to the classic concept of representing a model in mathematics before programming, but recognizes that some models are not reasonably expressed in mathematics.

Overall, our intent is to convey a sense of iterative work in which theory, model, and program are updated.

Even if we accept that a real system and truth exist, truth is multifaceted and subject to interpretation. Some of the differences may be only apparent when disciplines use different frames of reference for observing the same phenomena. Or they may be due to differences in levels of resolution (by analogy, the laws of thermodynamics or equilibrium statistical mechanics in physics). Still others are more fundamentally incommensurate. As an extreme, it is very difficult to compare between traditional Chinese medicine and mainstream medicine.

## Reality versus the Ideal

### Reality and Its Implications

Figure 4.1 represents a kind of ideal, but actual practice is, to say the least, sobering. In practice, models often exist only as computer programs,

---

[14] Reviewers of the report had differing views, ranging from "there is a lot more commonality than is generally realized" to "yes, there are distinctly different perspectives." The similarities and differences are discussed in Haack (2011, p.155ff.), in the chapter "The Same but Different."

[15] The role of sacred values is described persuasively by Scott Atran and Robert Axelrod (Atran, 2010; Atran and Axelrod, 2008). See also Čavojovà, 2018.

perhaps with some minimal overview in text explaining some aspects of the concepts behind them. Further, researchers do not have Figure 4.1 in mind. Rather, they often start by programming what they hope is a reasonable model, iterating until they feel satisfied—for good or bad reasons. This process is often decried for the lack of documentation, but pleading for documentation can be pedantic and lead to dubious bureaucratic "solutions." The better criticism is that

- the current process makes scientific reproduction, comparison, debate, review, and iteration difficult and rare.[16,17]
- the separation of "scientist" from "modeler" is puzzling.

Is a professor of anthropology really expected to master some large and opaque computer program to truly understand and review what it purports to describe? How much can that professor truly understand from just some overview essay?[18] And why is that professor not involved deeply in the modeling itself? In many fields, scientists or engineers do their own modeling. They may enlist specialists to do the more complicated programming after the fundamentals are solid, but until that point they (*or closely trusted graduate students*) are deeply involved.

---

[16] The embarrassing problem of models not actually being shared and reproduced was discussed in a conference panel (Uhrmacher et al., 2016). The panel's diagnosis pointed to both technical issues and protection of intellectual property. Levent Yilmaz, among others, has suggested directions for technical solutions (Yilmaz, 2012; Yilmaz and Ören, 2013).

[17] These problems have not gone unnoticed. Uri Wilensky and Bill Rand, for example, have proposed standards relating to replication and have illustrated their ideas in replicating an agent-based model (Wilensky and Rand, 2007).

[18] A special issue is that many anthropologists are skeptical about attempts to translate their knowledge into computer models. Some have an antipathy toward government projects related to national security or social interventions, which is rooted in anthropology's favoring cause-no-harm observation rather than intervention and a past history of anthropologists contributing to controversial government actions in Vietnam, counterterrorism torture activities, and the human-terrain-team functions in Iraq and Afghanistan. Still other concerns are rooted in the role that early anthropology played in justifying racist policies and eugenics in the nineteenth and twentieth centuries (Konner, 2003). Lawrence Kuznar discusses some of the moral dilemmas in his book on the field of anthropology (Kuznar, 2008). Wikipedia's article on Human Terrain Teams has extensive pointers to the original literature and media items debating the issues.

This is very different from "cooperating with" a graduate student from a modeling department (e.g., computer science, simulation, operations research) who needs an applied topic to use in demonstrating some method. Where is the graduate student's primary allegiance, and how deeply does the student get into the science?

**Moving Toward the Ideal**

It would be ridiculous to imagine that modelers and simulationists will "get religion" and adopt the construct of Figure 4.1 if it is interpreted to mean a linear process that moves in steps from rough theory to conceptual model to fully specified model to program. That would be fighting technology and might undercut the quality of modeling by deferring the creative parts. By programming from the outset and generating outputs to be compared with knowledge, the modeler can evolve his or her concepts quickly rather than comprehending "correctly" everything up front.[19] Nonetheless, there is much to be said for the ideal represented in Figure 4.1. We see some options for narrowing the gap between current reality and the ideal suggested.

Options
1. Live with what we are doing, but work harder (demand better documentation, etc.).
2. Strongly encourage use of modeling/programming systems that impose or strongly encourage rigorous and explicit procedures making the models comprehensible and "tight" to those familiar with the systems.[20]

---

[19] An analogy exists between this problem and the tension between the extremes of design-first programming and code-it-up-and-see programming in software development. The optimum is usually in between: "forcing" the modeler/programmer to do *some* explicit design first, then reviewing the concept but allowing early entry into the stage of rapid prototyping, followed by review and iteration. Careful discussion of such matters and risk-related trade-offs can be found in the work of software engineer Barry Boehm (Boehm and Hansen, 2000). Dangers in bootstrap-creative processes include poor design and a combination of conformation, anchoring, and motivational biases.

[20] As one example, the Discrete Event Simulation System (DEVS) promotes good practices within its domain (Zeigler et al., 2000). As another example, it is common now to use the Universal Modeling Language (UML) in object-oriented modeling (Blaha and Rumbaugh, 2005).

3.  Do the modeling initially in a high-level and comprehensible language.

4.  Do better and more explicit *conceptual* modeling by using a tool kit that includes, as appropriate, diagrams, input/output lists, level-of-resolution breakdowns, and key equations or pseudo-code.[21] Give up on mere mortals being able to understand implementing programs.

5.  Improve the comprehensibility and the norms for construction of computer models so that, with only moderate special training, the scientist's graduate student can comprehend, review, and debate efficiently. Many contemporary students already have significant programming skills.

Table 4.3 illustrates how such approaches might be compared. Doing a sounder comparison would require tightening the concepts and conducting experiments. Consider just some of the empirical questions:

- What kind of high-level depictions (diagrams, tables, pseudocode, etc.) *actually* speed and improve communication? Is there a distribution across people (e.g., with some people picking up diagram information faster and others learning better from tables)?
- How can content be effectively communicated with the various "high-level" methods (e.g., diagrams may or may not include information on algorithms).
- How many methods are necessary for the tool kit of someone attempting to do interdisciplinary work? The high-level methods for understanding agent-based models are likely always to be different from those for understanding system dynamical models and network models. Must all researchers be multilingual? How hard is that to achieve, if high-level versions exist for all?
- How much does the professor of anthropology really need to understand about model details before it is acceptable for him or her to trust graduate students to attend to additional details? In

---

[21] That might not be very different from what has been urged in agent-based modeling by Volker Grimm and associates (Grimm et al., 2010), but the tool kit would have to be broad enough to embrace other modeling styles (Uhrmacher et al., 2016; Yilmaz et al., 2007).

**Table 4.3**
**Comparing the Different Approaches**
*(Cell value shows notional assessment of the option (column) for achieving objective (row).)*

| | 1. Status quo (complex programs plus overview essay) | 2. Tighten by using rigorous procedures | 3. Use high-level language,[a] perhaps for operations or perhaps only for a specification model that runs | 4. Settle for comprehensible conceptual models and data sets | 5. Improve norms for documentation, coding, and standardization |
|---|---|---|---|---|---|
| Reproducibility | Very poor | Very good | Very good | Good | Good |
| Communication | Marginal to poor | Moderate | Very good | Good | Moderate |
| Peer review and debate | Very poor | Moderate | Very good | Good | Moderate |
| Composability | Poor, time intensive | Very good | Good, still difficult | Often good, often treacherous | Good |
| Reuse | Very poor | Very good | Good, perhaps with reprogramming | Good in multimodel approaches | Good |
| Ease of verification and tests pf internal validation | Very poor | Very good | Very good | N.A. | Good |

[a] Possible candidates: Some readers might think of Vensim, Analytica, Netica, or NetLogo, rather than C++, R, Fortran, or Python. Others might disagree (e.g., suggesting Python).

the natural sciences, scientists sometimes personally conduct experiments to affirm conclusions of their own laboratory; so also, anthropology professors sometimes go to the field personally to check on student observations.[22]

• If the ecology of applied model building, comparison, and iteration is good enough, how important are model details per se? Some argue that the related *process* of knowledge building and application is more important. Others are skeptical because model outputs are indeed used to inform decisions.

Such questions could be addressed in experiments and open publications, allowing the market to reach subsequent judgments. Within a given program, a narrow range of choices might be mandated for a degree of standardization (see Appendix A).

For all the approaches sketched in Table 4.3, there is also need for better education of consumers of model-based research and analysis. These consumers come from a range of backgrounds that often do not prepare them well for dealing with computationally intense analytic work. We see it as another empirical question: What mechanisms can mitigate these problems efficiently (e.g., one-week courses, a semester or one-year course, online courses, etc.)? Much experience exists but, to our knowledge, the effectiveness of existing methods has not been measured well.

If a more solid empirical basis existed for answering the questions above, then professional societies could be very useful in reviewing options, formulating and promulgating good practices, and educating scientists, modelers, and consumers of modeling and analysis. For example, societies could hold special workshops, tutorials, and short courses and issue sense-of-the-society reports. Many historical precedents exist for such activities.

---

[22] Members of the author team had personal experiences seeing such expressions of scientific integrity during their graduate school years—experiences with lasting effects on their own practices as researchers.

# CHAPTER FIVE

# Theory and Its Modeling

Having discussed the meta problem of better relating the three pillars of science in Chapter 3, let us now discuss selected challenges for theory and modeling.

## Assimilating Modeling Better into Social-Behavioral Science

An odd feature of today's social-behavioral (SB) research is that scientists and modelers are often different people in different departments.[1] One consequence has been that the scientists who have not yet bought into the power of computational science and simulation modelers in particular see themselves as specialists who apply their tools to such problems as arise without necessarily being impassioned by the science itself. In many other areas of science and engineering, the subject-matter people do their own modeling because (1) modeling is merely a tangible manifestation of the theory they are thinking about, rather than something different in kind; (2) being responsible for the applications, they want to fully understand the models and data brought to bear; and (3) they have found it possible to "pick up" the skills needed for at least the initial modeling during which core concepts are developed.[2]

---

[1]  In this discussion "modeling" refers to causal modeling of phenomena rather than use of statistical packages.

[2]  It is not unusual to rely on modeling and programming specialists when going beyond relatively simple prototypes. Neither Boeing, which counts on products with embedded

The worst-case version of social-behavioral modeling, which we have seen and heard others complain about, is when modelers speak only casually to scientists, go off and build their computer models, and then go back to the scientists asking them to "fill in the blanks" and estimate parameter values. The scientists may cooperate, but they loathe the situation because they believe that they should have been involved early, before the model's structure, character, and variables were determined.[3] Although we have seen better practice, this horror story is apparently not rare in social-behavioral work. The issues we raise here are not unique to SB modeling and simulation.

What options exist for closing the gap between scientists and modelers? With some exceptions, departments of social-behavioral research have not enthusiastically embraced computational modeling, but—if they do—how should they proceed? Possibilities include:

- Form cooperative projects in which the modelers are from other departments (e.g., a department of computer science, operations research, or even simulation per se).
- Develop modeling expertise in their own professors and graduate students.
- Take an interdisciplinary (or what some call a transdisciplinary) approach with close cooperation, so the scientists fully understand the model and the modelers thoroughly engage with the "real" science issues, not just building a model of some notional idealization.
- Pursue a hybrid approach.

DARPA and other government agencies can affect matters by, for example, demanding credible tight teaming in proposals. That may not be enough to move from multidisciplinary work to the kind of interdisciplinary work needed. In our experience, the best interdisciplin-

---

software, nor a team of high-energy physicists that counts on complex computer analysis to interpret faint data, can afford to depend on amateurish software.

[3]   This lament was first expressed to the senior author by former RAND colleague Kim Cragin, a cultural historian and counterterrorism expert.

ary work is sometimes characterized by participants coming to have a degree of disdain for specialist credentials and with everyone "getting in each other's knickers." The SBML approach described in Chapter 3 would encourage the cross-cutting.

## Assuring That Modeling Is Faithful to Subtleties of Theory

As mentioned in Chapter 2, a chronic problem with social-behavioral modeling has been that modelers often gloss over some of what the scientists regard as important. Many reasons for this exist: complexity of the real phenomena, shortcomings in current modeling and analysis tools, measurement difficulties, data availability, and hours in the day. Nonetheless, for the purposes of forward-leaning research, we see the following as especially important:

- A premium should exist for *causal* multivariate modeling even if statistical "models" are easier.
- Models should include the variables regarded as most important to understanding the phenomenon, whether those variables are "hard" or "soft."[4]
- Where proxies must be used when connecting with data, that should be a separate step that maintains visibility of the "real" variables.

  *Example*: Fear might be the real variable in some context; panic-laden speech or texting in social media might be *one* measurable indication of fear, but the extent of fear could be much greater than inferable from observation of speech and writing.

---

[4]  Soft variables can also be represented in statistical analysis and machine learning if one bothers to try, as illustrated in articles by computer scientist Lise Getoor and students (Farnadi et al., 2017). A recent book edited by Colette Faucher has a number of chapters describing efforts to make artificial intelligence agents that represent subtleties of culture (Faucher, 2018). The chapters include applications to, for example, health care, teaching Australian Aboriginal knowledge, enriching virtual characters, dealing with when beliefs and logic are in contradiction, and representing innovation.

- Models should include all variables necessary to differentiate important time sequences, such as scenarios.
  *Example*: Historical behavioral patterns may be quite different from future patterns in the wake of traumatic events.
  *Example*: One model may apply to a nationally representative population sample, but a very different model may apply to a subset of shadowy people with family ties to a particular ideology.
- Defining context may even require including troublesome variables, such as aspects of personal, cultural, and world-event histories,[5] and background cultural narratives.[6]
- Representing different perspectives must include confronting cases in which beliefs bear little relationship to scientific theory or logic (Čavojovà, 2018).
- Modeling should represent the dynamic nature of social-behavioral systems by recognizing, for example, the creation and disappearance of social units (not just strength of allegiance to them) and the creation and disappearance of macroscopic processes, flows, and concepts. In social-behavioral science, these are sometimes seen as emergent rather than "baked in." This relates to the idea of *variable structure simulations* (Uhrmacher and Zeigler, 1996; Mehlhase, 2014).

All of this could be a recipe for overcomplicated modeling that would be impossible to work with effectively. An overarching consideration is how to modularize and simplify when dealing with one or another level of detail and with one or another time scale. It will be necessary to make substantial advances in subjects such as multiresolution, multiperspective modeling and in coherently relating models that use different formalisms and levels of detail currently.[7] The last item

---

[5]   It is not always appropriate to assume Markov processes. Results may show what is called "path dependence."

[6]   Considerable literature exists on the importance of narratives and how to think about them (see Halverson et al., 2011; Eyre and Littleton, 2012; Corman, 2012).

[7]   An interesting aspect of multiscale work is the regularities that occur at different scales in organization, structure, and dynamics for diverse complex systems. See the review by Geoffrey West (West, 2017).

is particularly important because social science will continue to need a diversity of models. If the ultimate textbook is eventually written, it is unlikely to be a coherent masterpiece such as Euclid's, but rather a complex web connecting numerous theories and solutions.[8]

## Toward Multivariate Causal Models

As noted in Chapter 2 (in the section on "Need for Multivariate Causal Models"), a premium exists on causal models because they provide explanation and the ability to deal with circumstances different from those previously observed. Also, they are often necessary to aid in debate and decisionmaking because those making the decisions want to reason about cause-effect relationships, uncertainties, and conflicting considerations.

### Causality

The concept of causality is fundamental: It is built into the very structure of human languages and treated as a given in much scientific discussion. It is distinguished from mere correlation. Upon inspection, the concept is deep and the subject of considerable debate by philosophers, among others.[9] We see causal explanations as fundamental to understanding phenomena and to rational planning.

---

[8]  See page xv of the compelling book on this perspective by anthropologist and behavioral biologist Melvin Konner (Konner, 2003).

[9]  Mathematician Joseph Halpern distinguishes between "general causality" and "actual causality" (Halpern, 2016). Whether a relationship between two variables is causal depends on the model. A variable X may be a cause of a result R in model M1 but not model M2. Perhaps M2 is just "wrong" (its builder overlooked the role of X), but it may instead be that M2 represents a different but valid view of the world. Another theme in Halpern's book (especially Chapter 3) is that ascribing causality depends on assumptions about what is "normal." Such matters loom large in law when considering whether an individual or company is legally responsible for some problem.

Philosopher Nancy Cartwright also has a perceptive discussion of causality and its subtleties (Cartwright, 2004). She has famously written about how the laws of physics "lie" in that they pertain to idealized systems, not the real world. They inspire context-specific formulations, but those details of context are crucial—as they are in social science (Cartwright, 1983).

Admittedly, however, it is necessary to recognize the following:

1.  Effects often have multiple causes, with effects often being the result of nonlinear interactions among those causal factors. It seldom makes sense to ask whether B is caused by A, but rather whether A is one of the causal influences on B.
2.  Feedback effects are common in systems; they may be small and occur on relatively long time scales, but they can instead be large, immediate, or both. Because of feedback effects, it may be somewhat arbitrary whether one or another perspective of causality is more apt.
3.  Because of feedbacks, *simple* cause-effect relationships may be misleading, and it may be important to think about "balances" rather than simple cause-effect pairs and about different regions of the system's state space where relationships are different. This type of thinking is familiar in ecology, where populations rise and fall, sometimes dramatically, unless balances exist in predator-prey and other relationships.
4.  All of these items make the processes of verification and validation more challenging.

It is increasingly common today for even those researchers who are focused on data analysis to recognize the importance of discovering causal relationships rather than being satisfied with correlations. This has been the case for some years with econometricians (Angrist and Pischke, 2009), but is increasingly true more generally, due in part to the methods introduced by Judea Pearl for inferring causality from data. Pearl's seminal book on causality is the primary source for his thinking (Pearl, 2009b), but in a shorter paper he notes (Pearl, 2009a, p. 4):

> A useful demarcation line that makes the distinction between associational and causal concepts crisp and easy to apply, can be formulated as follows. An associational concept is any relationship that can be defined in terms of a joint distribution of observed variables, and a causal concept is any relationship that cannot be defined from the distribution alone. Examples of associational concepts are: correlation, regression, dependence, conditional inde-

pendence, likelihood, collapsibility, propensity score, risk ratio, odd ratio, marginalization, conditionalization, "controlling for," and so on. Examples of causal concepts are: randomization, influence, effect, confounding, "holding constant," disturbance, spurious correlation, faithfulness/stability, instrumental variables, intervention, explanation, attribution, and so on. The former can, while the latter cannot be defined in term of distribution functions.

This demarcation line is extremely useful in causal analysis for it helps investigators to trace the assumptions that are needed for substantiating various types of scientific claims. Every claim invoking causal concepts must rely on some premises that invoke such concepts; it cannot be inferred from, or even defined in terms of statistical associations alone.

To abstract from Pearl's description, we cannot really deal with issues such as influence, effect, confounding, holding constant, intervention, and explanation without causal models.

## Multivariate Aspects and Nonlinearity

Typically, good causal models will need to be multivariate because effects are not caused by individual discrete factors, but rather by combinations. The factors *may* contribute linearly, but often do not. In mathematical terms, to understand some effect $E$, a theory may characterize $E$ as a function of all of the contributing variables, i.e.,

$$E = E(X_1, X_2, \ldots X_n).$$

This is very different from a theory that postulates a series of discrete hypotheses, such as

$$E \sim X_1$$
$$E \sim X_3$$
$$E \sim X_5,$$

i.e., that $E$ should increase with increasing values of $X_1$ and $X_3$ and with decreasing values of $X_5$. If one were to test this type of theory empirically, one would use a linear regression in the three variables and look to see if the coefficients of the three variables were sizable and statistically significant. If the empirical coefficients proved statistically insignificant, it would seem that the hypotheses were falsified and that the three variables were not important to $E$. It might be, however, that the three variables are significant, as are the omitted variables $X_2$, $X_4$, $X_5$, etc., but that the functional form is nonlinear and—for the conditions of testing—the effects of the three variables are being obscured. For example, suppose that the functional form is such that for large values of $X_4$ (the only ones for which data exists), $E$ does not change with $X_1$, $X_3$, and $X_5$.[10]

## Dealing Routinely with Uncertainty

To represent the richness of the science, Chapter 2 proposed distinguishing among validity for description, explanation, postdiction, exploratory analysis and coarse prediction, and classic prediction. A related issue is how to think about model-based analysis. When uncertainties abound, different attitudes about analysis are needed. This is especially true where *deep* uncertainty exists. In early years, system analysts used the terms "real uncertainty" or "scenario uncertainty" to mean the same thing. An example of *non*-deep uncertainty would be playing the game of craps in an honest casino. Results are uncertain, but the odds are well understood. Even stock-market investments can be regarded as straightforward for the long term if one believes that the statistics of the past are roughly right looking forward. In contrast,

> Deep uncertainty is the "condition in which analysts do not know or the parties to a decision cannot agree upon (1) the appropriate

---

[10] As an example, suppose United Nations forces intervene to stabilize some troubled country. The extent of foreign aid may be irrelevant to results because intervention forces are insufficient to provide even a modicum of security or because the government being assisted is so deeply corrupt as to divert nearly all aid to private accounts. As a contrasting example, if the size of the intervention force were large enough, adding still more forces would probably not improve prospects (and might even reduce them because of reactions to foreign presence), while more economic and political aid might prove valuable. Both examples illustrate effects of nonlinearity, as discussed in a volume reviewing social science for intervention operations (Davis, 2011).

models to describe interactions among a system's variables, (2) the probability distributions to represent uncertainty about key parameters in the models, and/or (3) how to value the desirability of alternative outcomes." (Lempert et al., 2003)

We discuss analysis under deep uncertainty in Chapter 7. The recommended analysis, however, requires models that will support exploratory work that considers uncertainties in many dimensions (an n-dimensional uncertainty space, or scenario space). If models can be expressed as rather simple formulas, this is not a problem. With more complicated models, such as the simulations often used to investigate behavior of complex systems, the usual approaches to model design make such uncertainty analysis very difficult or impossible. The curse of dimensionality proves overwhelming, and the tendency is then to fall back to using the model for only a few cases.

As computer scientist Steven Bankes discussed in a seminal 1990s paper, it follows that we need to design models and platforms differently to go about what he called exploratory modeling (Bankes, 1993). By that time, that had already begun to happen (Davis and Winnefeld, 1983), but in subsequent years numerous developments proved feasibility and practicality. Many different methods and mechanisms have been used, but a cross-cutting principle is that one needs simpler models (fewer independent variables) for exploration and richer models to go more deeply into specific and contextually subtle issues as needed. This may require multiresolution modeling or multiresolution families of models (Davis, 2003).

## Going Beyond Simulation: Using a Portfolio of Modeling Methods

Social-behavioral scientists already use numerous analytical methods that can be seen as types of models.[11] Often, however, modelers think immediately of simulation modeling—i.e., of modeling that

---

[11] Metaphors can be seen as models (Konner, 2015). So also, when people refer to sensemaking they are essentially constructing models (Madsbjerg, 2017).

generates predicted behaviors of the system over time.[12] This includes system-dynamic, agent-based, and other commonly used methods. The ambition of being able to simulate system behaviors and thereby inform options for influencing those systems has been an ideal for many years.[13]

Despite our enthusiasm for and experience with simulation, it is preferable for a social-behavioral research program to use a wider portfolio of models and tools. We mention a few of them here: (1) analytical models (think of them, roughly, as formula models), (2) equilibrium or steady-state models that require computational solution, (3) knowledge-based simulation, (4) game theory, and (5) human exercises.

1. Analytical models abound in social sciences. They include classic economic models based on rational actors, textbook-level game theory, and epidemiological models (e.g., the SIR model that focuses on the susceptible, infected, and recovered classes of individual in a population affected by a disease).[14]

2. Equilibrium or steady-state models are important in physics, chemistry, and physiology, among other subjects.[15]

3. "Knowledge-based simulation" (KBSim) is not well known but was designed for "Beyond What-If Questions?" A model can be designed as a rule-based simulation and then used not to ask

---

[12] The dictionary definition of "simulation" is broader, but associating simulation with the generation of behavior over time fits the most common usage in the modeling and analysis communities.

[13] Examples include early work on system dynamics (Forrester, 1963), the later work of Dietrich Dörner, better known in Europe than in the United States (Dörner, 1997), and agent-based work on artificial societies (Epstein and Axtell, 1996).

[14] SIR models refer to susceptible individuals, infected individuals, and recovered individuals. Some versions can be solved analytically; some require numerical solution.

A number of authors have written on how to weaken assumptions about strict rationality. Some have come from anthropology (Hruschka, 2010), some from economics (Della Vigna and Malmender, 2006), and some from such other fields as political science. An interesting example is modeling decisionmaking based on initial "rational" thinking, followed by heuristics that represent subsequent results of social interactions (Rahimian and Jadbabaie, 2016).

[15] See related comments by Herbert Simon (Simon, 1990).

about a result (What if . . . ?) but rather "Under what circumstances will the result be ___?" This depends on "backward chaining" inference, as is possible with the programming language *Prolog*.[16]

4.  Game theory models and related simulation are often powerful, sometimes for finding optimal strategies in many domains. Game theory methods can then be compared with those of more descriptive models, highlighting aspects of bounded rationality and other real-world considerations (Pita et al., 2010).

5.  Human exercises are a form of modeling. Consider a military war game or a commercial version of a war game. Players have a finite set of permitted moves; the "rulebook" (or an adjudication team) determines the results of the various player moves and other events. The game proceeds over time. Such human-in-the-loop simulations often have major advantages over usual computer simulations because the humans are less constrained, more creative, and ultimately more complex (with multiple factors affecting their actions, including competition, emotion, and judgments about their adversaries). To the extent that social-behavioral modeling sometimes suffers by being inadequately realistic, gaming would be one mechanism for complementing and/or testing.[17]

Figure 5.1 shows just some of the many modeling types that are mentioned. The left side of the figure comes from an NRC report; all of the methods shown are quantitative. We have added boxes on the right to remind us of different forms. These lists are by no means complete.

---

[16] DARPA's programs in artificial intelligence sponsored work of this character in earlier years (Rothenberg, 1989; Rothenberg and Narain, 1994).

[17] Human gaming is a broadly applicable method (Schwabe, 1994) used in many domains, including business (Herman and Frost, 2009) and domestically oriented policy analysis. A recent professional-society workshop was devoted to war gaming (Pournelle, 2016) and its relationship to modeling and analysis (Davis, 2017). Readers may be more familiar with recreational games, including massively multiplayer online games (MMOGs) (see Zacharias et al., 2008). The concept of "serious games" is now well recognized (Zyda, 2007; National Research Council, 2010).

**Figure 5.1**
**A Similarity Network of Modeling Methods**

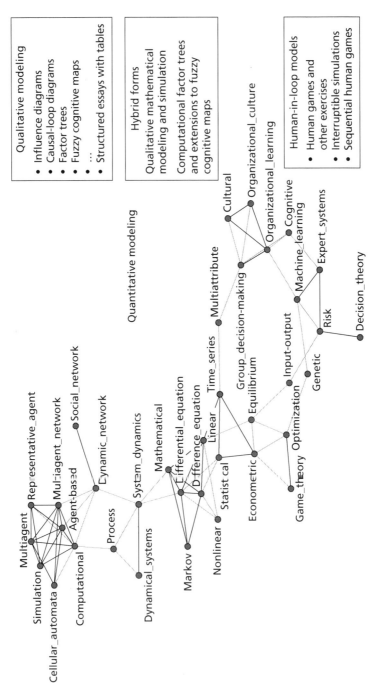

SOURCE: Adapted from NRC report (Zacharias et al., 2008, p. 93).

## Toward Greater Generality, Synthesis, and Coherence

### Issues

Perhaps the biggest challenge for representing social-behavioral science in models is that current theories tend to be fragmented and to lack the coherence needed for modeling. An objective, then, is to encourage research to integrate and synthesize, to move toward clumps of more general and coherent theory. This should cross boundaries not only of current social and behavioral sciences, but also neurophysiology. Some of the obstacles include economic incentives, academic incentives (e.g., will the work be valued by those who vote on tenure decisions?), and the well-known difficulties of interdisciplinary work.[18] Let as assume, however, that these can be overcome (if the incentives exist in the form of exciting challenges and research grants). Doing so is outside the scope of this report, but subsequent sections discuss issues of scale and perspective, reconciling models across type, formalism, and scale; synthesis by putting the pieces together; synthesis through multiresolution modeling; integration by transformation function; and coordination rather than integration.

### Scale and Perspective

One challenge here is the need for models or model families that deal with multiple scales of detail and/or alternative perspectives (e.g., individual-centric versus culture-centric), which are sometimes called in the literature (Davis and Bigelow, 1998; Yilmaz et al., 2007) multiresolution, multiperspective models (MRMPM).[19] The phrase "or model families" is important because building alternative resolution levels into a single model can be useful to a point, but produces an overly

---

[18] Some unusual examples of cross-cutting work involve neuroeconomics (Zak, 2012) and an anthropologist's study showing how biological, economic, and family circumstances work together to cause lifelong problems for children (Lende, 2012). Psychologists have studied within-individual variability of personality, drawing on a biologically based theoretical framework (Read et al., 2017). An early example used system dynamics to consider international issues related to climate, trade, and globalization (Lofdahl, 2001).

[19] In some literature, multiresolution modeling refers to modeling only at a detailed level, but then generating *displays* at lower resolution. That is not our meaning.

complicated model if too many options exist. It is then better to have separate models for different levels (or perspectives) *and to have well-established relationships among them*, as in integrated hierarchical variable resolution models (IHVR) (Davis and Hillestad, 1993).

Progress requires that the relationships among model types be better understood, more rigorous, and more convenient. It is rather striking at this point (2017) that little work has been done to relate system dynamics and agent-based models except in "stapled together" versions of multimodels or in laudable individual studies to see how such models compare (Rahmandad and Sterman, 2008).[20]

Where is the analogue to the relationship between statistical molecular physics and thermodynamics? Or the analogue to understanding the phases and phase transitions of CAS as we understand phase transitions in fluids? Also, why is it that we have difficulty knowing which social science theories are merely equivalent representations and which are somehow incommensurate? Why is it that the usual assumption is that agents are microscopic and that system dynamics is highly aggregated and idealized?

Speculatively, might we not expect that in-depth theoretical work using both agent-based models (ABMs) and system dynamic (SD) models in a particular problem area would lead to interesting conclusions or suggestions. Possibilities include:

1.   Revised SD models that have more structure to reflect macroscopically the consequences of factions and perhaps better representation of "frictional effects" due to microscopic interactions being less than perfectly efficient.
2.   Stochastic SD models that represent some matters with probability distributions with basis in ABM-level work, including multimodal distributions.
3.   ABMs with more aggregate-level agents.

---

[20] Considerable information and inspiration on such matters can be drawn from biology, as in discussions by Jessica Flack about multiscale phenomena in nature—e.g., pigtailed macaque social organization and management (Flack, 2012). Flack also has a remarkable discussion about how moral systems in primates can be seen as an aggregation of building-block systems (Flack and de Waal, 2000; Flack et al., 2005).

Consider Figure 5.2, a schematic of a multiresolution model or family of models. One can choose to work at any of the levels indicated, choosing inputs and outputs appropriately. In designing the structure of each, however, one might look to models of greater and lesser resolution for guidance. Similarly, if setting parameter values at a given level, one might use information from exercising models of greater or lesser resolution to help do so. To be somewhat less abstract, suppose one is building and tuning a model at the intermediate level. The tuning should be consistent with credible aggregate information from the next level up (e.g., the *sentiment of the crowd*). It should also be consistent with what can be understood from exercising the lowest-level (highest-resolution) model. For example, if the intermediate model only recognizes two factions even though dozens exist microscopically, those two factions should be seen as aggregations of smaller ones. Would the aggregation be simple or the result of influence weighting, or what?[21]

The goal in working with multiresolution families and related data should be to build self-consistent models at different levels—i.e., models that make the best use of all relevant knowledge. This is in contrast with imagining that macrolevel models and their parameter values should be derived *solely* bottom-up. The pure bottom-up notion, popular in Defense Department viewgraphs over roughly fifty years, is fundamentally flawed. As an analogue, thermodynamics is now understandable and derivable from molecular-level statistical mechanics, but the values of important macroscopic parameters must still be determined empirically—in part because the theoretical work necessarily makes approximations that are not always accurate, much less precise. Further, the theoretical derivations have often been strongly informed by knowing what thermodynamics-level laws are empirically valid (i.e., theoretical work has benefited from empirical hints).[22]

---

[21] This issue is discussed as an example of how moving from a qualitative model to a computational model requires specifying algorithms that require empirical information, not just logic (Davis and O'Mahony, 2013). In the meantime, recognizing alternative logics can be useful for uncertainty analysis.

[22] A reviewer commented that this paragraph illustrates that theories and models in physics are more analogous than sometimes realized. In particular, they come about from a combination of bottom-up and top-down reasoning and observation, rather than a strictly

**Figure 5.2**
**Multiresolution Models**

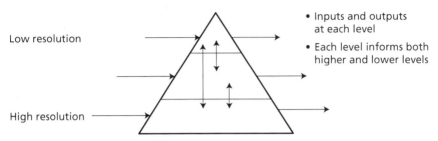

Low resolution

High resolution

- Inputs and outputs at each level
- Each level informs both higher and lower levels

SOURCE: Adapted from National Research Council, 1997, and Davis and Bigelow, 1998.
RAND *RR2208-5.2*

If Figure 5.2 envisions representing phenomena at different resolutions, an entirely separate issue is representing phenomena through different perspectives.

In physics, an example might be describing motion in a rotating coordinate system rather than a rectilinear coordinate system. In that case, the alternative perspectives or representations are equivalent. In contrast, in social-behavioral modeling, we may be concerned about representing different worldviews, scientific frameworks, or narratives (e.g., an individual-centric framework or a culture-centric framework). These may or may not be mere translations of each other.

### Reconciling Models Across Type, Formalism, Resolution, and Perspective

It may seem incongruous to have competing theories and models. Surely, one must be *right* (or none of them). Or perhaps not. This is a deep issue in the social sciences, but not uniquely there (think of the wave-particle duality of quantum mechanics). To be sure, some models may be falsified and discarded; some may possibly be "valid" but are found to be not useful. Nonetheless, we will often find ourselves with competing models and no clear relationships among them. Improving on this state

---

deductive approach starting with first principles. Further, the parameter values of the laws of physics (e.g., Maxwell's equations) depend on *context*. It is not just social scientists who are sensitive to contextual matters!

of affairs is nontrivial, but in-depth study might indicate any of the following:

1. The models are separately valid but describe different facets of the system.
2. The models are separately valid and equivalent, describing the same phenomena with different terminology or formalisms, or through different lenses (recall rectangular and rotating coordinate systems in physics).
3. The models may apply to different contexts (i.e., applying to different portions of the system's state space).
4. The models disagree, perhaps with some overlap, and ultimately represent conflicting frameworks that may or may not be resolvable.

What can be done when we encounter such issues? We discuss some possibilities in the following subsections.

### Synthesis by Putting the Pieces Together

In some instances, the chaos of conflicting social science theories is probably due to disciplinary and personal parochialism. It *should* then be possible to achieve qualitative synthesis with a conceptual model that includes all the variables (factors) highlighted by the competing theories, acknowledging that behaviors will be due to all of these variables and attempting to understand the larger function that describes behavior. When using such a general theory, different factors can be seen naturally as being more and less significant to an outcome as a function of context. A decade ago, arguments about "the" root cause of terrorism were highly fragmented in this way (Figure 5.3), with separate researchers studying such diverse causes as deprivation, insanity, and nationalism. A DoD-sponsored study by RAND accomplished a *qualitative* synthesis using the factor-tree methodology (Figure 5.4), which makes it easy to understand that different factors are more important in different cases (Davis and Cragin, 2009). Thus, it is foolish to argue about which of the "theories" in Figure 5.3 is correct (although some have been falsified, as with research showing that terrorists are not particularly afflicted with mental illness). Rather, the more general qualitative

**Figure 5.3**
**Starting with a Grab-Bag of Competing Theories for the Root**
**Cause of Terrorism**

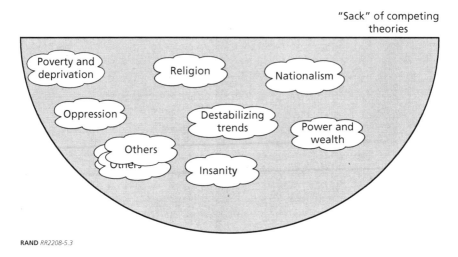

theory of Figure 5.4 sharpens the meaning of "Well, what matters most depends on context." A later study sought to qualitatively validate a factor tree for public support of terrorism. It corroborated this expectation by showing that the relative significance of factors varied greatly for cases involving al Qaeda, the Turkish PKK (Kurdistan Workers' Party), the Nepalese Maoists, and the Taliban (Davis et al., 2012). In pictorial terms, this was indicated with factor trees (akin to Figure 5.4) with some arrowed lines being much thicker than others.

### Synthesis Through Multiresolution Theory

In some instances, a multiresolution theory may allow synthesis. It is likely that a properly designed system dynamical theory should often be consistent with and be more useful in analysis than the appropriately *aggregated* results of relatively microscopic, bottom-up, agent-based modeling theory. Many of the arguments for why this will not be true are flawed because of simplistic versions of both types of theory. A theory expressed in systems dynamics, for example, need not assume homogeneous systems and may instead recognize a number of distinguishable macroscopic entities. So also, a correct aggregate depiction of

**Figure 5.4**
**Synthesis by Putting Pieces Together**

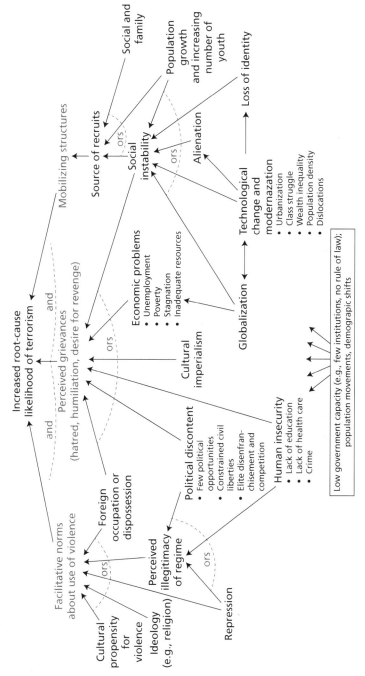

a phenomenon (i.e., a system dynamics theory motivated from experiments with an agent-based model) will typically not assume simple averaging. Rather, the aggregate-level consequences of more microscopic complexity may be reflected in, for example, (1) coefficients and terms reflecting mean consequences of complex nonlinear interactions and (2) a stochastic model in which key variables are represented by distribution functions.[23]

So also, a correct aggregate model might represent alternative pathways corresponding to alternative emergent phenomena in a bottom-up view. Is this so fundamentally different from chemistry theory that recognizes phase transitions and uncertainties about when transitions will occur (e.g., by recognizing uncertainties about whether appropriate catalysts will exist or whether adequate stirring exists in circumstances that might otherwise see phase changes)? Although it is common to associate the emergence phenomena of complex adaptive systems with systems having sentient agents, similar nonlinear phase-changing emergent phenomena have long been observed in physical systems (Bar-Yam, 1997; Nicolis and Prigogine, 1977).

### Integration by Transformation Functions
In some instances, separate theories may be consistent and mutually understandable if merely we know the transformation functions (a Rosetta stone would be a metaphor). Just as a physicist can move readily from a rectangular to a rotating coordinate system, it may also be possible for some social science theories to be mapped into one another well. The metaphor here might be of computer languages. Initially, programs written in functional versus procedural languages might seem incommensurate, but they might both represent the same phenomena equivalently.

As one well-known example, suppose that a first theory of decision assumes a rational actor and expresses itself in mathematics. Suppose a

---

[23] It is common to use stochastic models microscopically and then assume that more aggregate models should be deterministic. That is frequently not the case, however. As a simple example, aggregate models of weather may predict tomorrow's probability of rain, snow, ice, or no precipitation. When tomorrow's temperatures may be anywhere in the range of 20–35 degrees, we do not want forecasters to tell us "the" prediction by saying, "Oh, tomorrow will be rainy at 33 degrees."

second theory is expressed only in essay format and refers to religiosity, passions, and allegiances (more of a norms-based theory). When applying these to the question of why an individual becomes a suicide bomber in the name of jihad, it may at first appear that the rational-actor theory is simply wrong. It can be argued, however, that the action is rational if merely one uses the terrorist's utility function, which emphasizes neither individual survival nor materialism but instead gives great weight to the jihadi *cause* on behalf of "brother Muslims" worldwide, the religious obligation for jihad, and the conclusion that only suicide bombing works as a tactic because jihadis lack conventional power. In this case, the rational-actor formalism can be made to work—explaining terrorist choices as to when and whether to use suicide bomber tactics. The trick is transforming "soft" discussion of motivations into the mathematical language of rational-actor theory. Economists sometimes refer to this extension of theory as allowing for altruistic utilities.[24]

In other cases, no such transformation is sensible. Some individuals, for example, behave in ways that *should* be considered irrational. Attempting to infer a utility function by revealed preferences is then problematic because no *stable* utility function exists, perhaps because of temporary effects of emotion, exhaustion, or illness (National Research Council, 2014, pp. 335–337).

### Coordination Rather Than Integration

In some instances, it is almost certain that alternative social science theories will remain incommensurate to at least a significant degree. For example, in modeling the leader of an adversary nation, a political-science model might look at crude power-balance considerations, a cognitive model might attempt to represent the results of the adversary's reasoning "as though" the reasoning was intendedly rational but affected by misperceptions, and a psychiatric model might draw on the leader's history from the womb through adulthood to anticipate

---

[24] See, for example, Berrebi and Lakdawalla, 2007; and Berrebi, 2009. The potential for being able to map between seemingly different theories is described in a companion paper (Nyblade et al., 2017) drawing highlights from the theoretical literature in social-behavioral science. The importance of addressing the *adversary's* perceptions and values dates back at least to Robert Jervis (Jervis, 1976).

behavior.[25] Some synthesis-by-knocking-heads-together would be possible, but it is unclear how far such synthesis could proceed. It might be better merely to recognize the different models, characterize where one might be particularly better than others, or allow decisionmakers to synthesize in their own heads, drawing on information that is not contained in the separate models (e.g., impressions from personal meetings or special intelligence).

## Improving Scientific Practices

A reality frequently discussed informally is that social-behavioral computational modeling suffers in part because it often does not exhibit classic characteristics of good science such as reproducibility, comprehensibility, peer review, and iteration. Even when counterexamples appear to exist, questions arise about whether "reproducibility" amounts only to running a computer code and verifying that, yes, if we run the same model we get the same results (no, that is not what reproducibility means in science). Also, when one group adapts aspects of another group's computer code, how much does that say about how well the groups understood and critically assessed claims about the basic science? Such issues are among the reasons for the less-than-overwhelming acceptance of computational social science in the broader scientific community.

The issue of reproducibility has been discussed seriously in professional settings, as in a conference working group organized by Adelinde Uhrmacher of the University of Rostock (Uhrmacher et al., 2016). Some of the problems identified relate to the perceived need to protect intellectual property and are unlikely to go away or be easily resolved. Other problems are at least potentially amenable to solution with improved methods and technology, as discussed by Levent Yilmaz and Tuncer Ören of Auburn and Toronto universities (Yilmaz and Ören, 2013).

---

[25] The U.S. Central Intelligence Agency (CIA) has long done behavioral profiling of foreign leaders, which has included psychiatric interpretations (Post, 2008). Simple cognitive modeling has been applied to Saddam Hussein (Davis, 1994) and, more recently, to North Korea (Davis, 2017). One well-developed strand of political-science modeling stems from the work of Bruce Bueno de Mesquita (Bueno de Mesquita, 1983; Bueno de Mesquita, 2010; also see Abdollahian et al., 2006).

In our view, the problems of comprehensibility, peer review, and the like have to some extent been denied by computational social scientists because they are wedded to computer programming and see it as a natural fact of life that such programs are not very comprehensible to nonprogrammers (why should they be?). Be that as it may, we anticipate replicability crises in computational social science.

As suggested earlier, it should also be a major goal to ensure that models are comprehensible and debated in depth by social-behavioral scientists.

# CHAPTER SIX

# Experimentation

Many other challenges exist for experimentation. Here we discuss a selected number meriting special attention.

## Theory-Informed Experimentation

As discussed throughout our report, it is particularly important—for the purposes of DARPA's efforts—to increase the emphasis on multivariate *causal* theory. This implies that an experimental effort (whether empirical or computational) should be theory-informed if it is to be useful in evaluating or influencing theory.

Mathematically, some of the problems are due to the data analysis requiring 1:n mappings (i.e., disaggregation). The only easy approach assumes uniformity, but that may be misleading.[1] Another fundamental problem is missing data. If scientists know that the strength of a phenomenon depends on various contextual matters, but information about that context is missing in the empirical data, what then?

What does it mean to suggest theory-informed approaches? This is a general problem in science, but one that has more specific implications in social-behavioral work. It also means confronting some disagreements of paradigm. Many data analysts believe empirical analysis should be pure, untainted by theory. Others believe that the focus should be on that which can be measured well, even if other variables

---

[1]  As an example, if the average appeal of ISIS propaganda to teenagers is very low, what should be assumed about the *distribution* of risk-taking propensities among teenagers?

might be of interest. Still others are strongly concerned about not allowing more variables than can be shown to have statistical significance from finite data. A theory-informed approach, then, may encounter resistance. We offer three observations here.[2]

### Urging a Theory-Informed Approach Is Not Radical

First, focusing on testing and improving theory is not really so radical. Indeed, one of the most cited of statisticians, George Box, long ago argued forcefully for using empirical analysis *to test and inform theory improvement, rather than to infer some "pure" empirical expressions.* He discussed such matters in a paper entitled "Statistics for Discovery" (Box, 2000), which suggests the kind of tight loop between causal theory and empirical data highlighted in Figure 3.1. Political scientist Philip Schrodt, in a well-known paper, identified "seven deadly sins of contemporary quantitative political analysis" (Schrodt, 2013), some of which would clearly be mitigated by informing the regression specification with theory, if such theory exists.[3] The theory we have in mind here will typically be causal, multivariate, and perhaps systemic in character, rather than in the nature of a hypothesis or even a linear sum of discrete hypotheses.

### To Inform with Theory Is Not to Impose a Theory

Second, it is important to recognize that a "theory-informed approach" should not undercut empirical work by *imposing* a theory. A theory-informed approach should be one that "gives theory a chance" by ensuring that the specification used to define the statistical analysis includes terms representing theory, or fragments of theory, while also including terms of a more common nature (e.g., terms linear in the easy-to-measure variables, an error term, and perhaps one or more interaction terms). If the theory term proves to have significant statistical explana-

---

[2]   The theory-empiricism divide has been a concern for many years. An interesting and perceptive discussion of it in the domain of political science occurred in a workshop of the National Science Foundation (see particularly Appendices B and C) (Political Science Program, 2002).

[3]   Although we merely mention the point to avoid digression on a contested point, we take the view that empirical analysis is never theory-free as sometimes claimed. For example, the statistician referring to Occam's razor and using linear regression is making assumptions about the actual nature of the phenomenon.

tory capability, that will tend to confirm the theory; if that does not occur, then nothing is lost: The result can then be a regression relationship with no obvious relationship to theory. This approach has been called *motivated metamodeling* in past work and has been used in a number of studies (Bigelow and Davis, 2003). Note that in this approach it should be possible to have routine competition between data-driven and theory-informed approaches.

## Connections Exist with Multiresolution Modeling

Third, we see a strong relationship between the challenges here (informing data collection and analysis) and the need for multiresolution modeling as described earlier. Figure 6.1 shows a notional relationship among variables that might be suggested by theory: The effect E in the phenomenon of interest is "caused" by more than a dozen variables (m, n, . . . z). If the experimentalist is told to think about fifteen independent variables when analyzing data, the response might be to quit talking to the theorist. However, theory is actually claiming that only m, n, and o have important effects. Lower-level variables manifest their effects through them. Can m, n, and o be estimated well enough to make comparisons with observations of E? Note that in the hypothetical theory, some causal connections are discounted (the dashed lines), some are stronger than others (darker), and some might be ignored for approximate work except to require the inclusion of an error term. Unfortunately, most current software for generating influence diagrams, causal-loop diagrams, fuzzy cognitive maps, etc., does not allow making such visible distinctions, even though they are natural to point out in looking at data.[4] As a result, the diagrams are often far more complicated than they need to be.

Relationships vaguely like those of Figure 6.1 occur in many domains. The intermediate variables m, n, and o may be akin to, say, frictions or efficiencies. Ultimately, they might be complex functions of lower-level causal variables predictable in principle, but—as a practical

---

[4] An example was using factor trees to interpret information in case studies of public support for terrorism. As expected, the same factor tree applied in different contexts *but* with the factors having different relative strengths (Bigelow and Davis, 2003). Those factors could also change over time as the government and insurgents sought new ways to attract support.

**Figure 6.1**
**Multiresolution Modeling and Variables of Empirical Analysis**

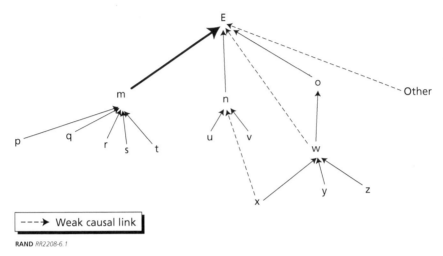

RAND RR2208-6.1

matter—they have to be empirically measured. An example in behavioral work might be the "fixation of belief" in psychology, a concept suggested by Charles S. Peirce in the late nineteenth century (Peirce, 1877). A corollary of this example is that empirical work will require *simplified theory* if it is to be theory informed in a realm of difficult-to-measure variables. In the social-behavioral realm, methods such as factor trees and fuzzy cognitive maps may prove useful in providing such simplified models.[5]

## Other Issues

### Estimating Difficult-to-Measure Variables

Giving increased emphasis to causal theory implies the need for empirical work to address variables that are soft and difficult or impossible to measure. The difficulties are well known to social scientists generally

---

[5] Examples of both are included in articles of a special issue (volume 14, no. 1) of the *Journal of Defense Modeling and Simulation* (Davis and O'Mahony, 2017; and Osoba and Kosko, 2017).

(Nyblade et al., 2017), but "doing better" is more easily demanded than accomplished. A rethinking is necessary about what should be accomplished and how. It is also imperative that the data sought be "close to the ground" in many instances or else important subtleties will be lost, a point made by Richard Davis, among others (R Davis, 2016).

### Speed, Tailoring

It is predictable that compelling reasons will exist for fast analysis to support judgments and decisions in minutes or days, rather than months and years. Further, as occurs after terrorist events or warning of terrorist attacks, it will sometimes be necessary to quickly collect and process data tailored to the particular issue and context. The process of assessing needs, designing data or experiments, collecting, and analyzing may again need to be remarkably fast by the standards of past years and ordinary processes. Technology will probably permit this if the methods and data structures are in place.

### Joint Planning for Empirical and Computational Experimentation

Accepting that the three pillars supporting science are theory and both empirical and computational observation and experimentation, it follows that planning of experiments should change radically so that both mechanisms are used and that priorities for both are set jointly. This may be a phased process:

1. In the first phase, empirical information is needed to test the approximate validity of the models. Since only limited empirical information is plausible, it will be necessary to establish priorities. Modelers will often know where their models are most and least solid. For example, if the model generates phase diagrams of the system showing context regions with different degrees of stability, the modelers may be far more confident that the different phases exist than where their boundaries are. "Tipping

points" may be inherently empirical, but theory and models may predict where to look for them.[6]

2.  In the second phase, after models have been shown to have reasonable validity for exploration, they may suggest contexts that would be especially favorable for a contemplated intervention. Empirical data might then be crucial to check results in more detail than before, because a degree of fine-tuning is necessary and/or because even model predictions depend sensitively on some variables that can be measured.

Concepts for how to go about this type of thing are well developed in certain domains of engineering, where organizations ultimately depend on the model to inform their decisions and therefore must use testing efficiently to validate their model.[7] Some nice examples exist also in social science, as in work using empirical data on primate conflict and Monte Carlo modeling to infer decisionmaking strategies being used, a kind of inductive game theory (DeDeo et al., 2010). Another example involves a data-driven, agent-based modeling framework (with an embedded theory of consumer choice) in connection with machine learning used to understand the adoption of solar energy (Zhang et al., 2016).

It is well to end this section by observing that if the *process* of knowledge building and sharing is often more important than the individual artifacts (i.e., individual versions of particular models), then attention must be paid to the knowledge-building ecology and the health of interactions among researchers and analysts, who *use* models and simulation but are ultimately responsible for providing insights and advice and for building cumulative comprehensible knowledge. To illustrate

---

[6]  Agent-based modeling in economics, for example, may highlight instabilities that may (or may not) lead to market collapses, such as occurred in the late 1990s and in 2007–2008 (Bookstaber, 2017).

[7]  As one example, when the U.S. Air Force developed the Peacekeeper intercontinental ballistic missile (ICBM), it recognized that establishing the intended accuracy and reliability empirically would have required very large numbers of test flights at varied ranges, azimuths, and so on. Instead, it focused on validating a model by using a moderately small number of flight tests (~20) (see U.S. General Accountability Office, 1989).

the point, anyone responsible for policy analysis that makes use of modeling is aware that "the" models used in a given analysis are seldom off-the-shelf. Rather, the analytic team knows how to craft variants of model and data suitable to addressing the particular questions at issue. Such at-the-time crafting is a distinctive feature of first-rate analytic organizations.

## New Sources and New Technology

One of the most important developments in the last decade bearing on social-behavioral science is the burgeoning of new data sources, such as those associated with social media (e.g., Twitter, Facebook) and what is just beginning in the era of the Internet of Everything (IoE). Social media data and IoE data streams are current examples of newer data streams in the growing data ecosystem. They augment and improve on traditional sources of behavioral data like ethnographies and surveys. Other sources include cellular data records, satellite imaging, GPS traces, smartgrid usage reports, point-of-sale transactions data, and health records.

Such data streams are accessible singly, in curated platform bundles from iOS, Android, Twitter, and the National Oceanic and Atmospheric Administration, or even from third-party data aggregation and embellishment services. Most of these new data streams offer new and nonoverlapping perspectives on human behaviors. The data ecosystem will continue to grow, motivated by the need for data to inform accountability or intelligence functions. Access to these streams will also most likely continue to grow, subject to financial, legal, or policy constraints.

In parallel, machine learning and related versions of artificial-intelligence research have advanced greatly as described in a companion paper (Osoba and Davis, forthcoming). This includes the development of methods for fusing data sets, methods for combining knowledge and models, methods for rendering new data streams more behaviorally informative, or methods for directly modeling social behavior. These artificial intelligence/machine learning AI/ML developments, com-

**Table 6.1**
**New Methods and Technology in a Recent Review of Sensemaking**

| Citation | Subject |
| --- | --- |
| Elson et al., 2014 | Frameworks and methods for data collection |
| Brashears and Sallach, 2014 | Modeling techniques |
| Ryan, 2014 | N-dimensional visualization for big data |
| Irvine, 2014 | Transforming heterogeneous data into sociocultural patterns |
| Sanfillipo et al., 2014 | Discovering behavioral patterns |
| Fricker et al., 2014 | Effects of visualization and data analysis on user understanding of phenomena |
| Gabbay, 2014 | Distinctions among processing for forecasting, understanding, and detecting |
| Lustick, 2014 | Visualizations for understanding |
| Sliva, 2014 | Methods to assist course of action development |
| Yost, 2014 | Visualization |
| Elsaesser et al., 2014 | Computational models for forecasting |

NOTE: All citations refer to chapters in Egeth et al. (2014).

bined with many items in the MITRE report of results of DoD's ear-lier Human, Social and Culture Behavior Modeling (HSCB) program (Egeth et al., 2014), are highly relevant. Table 6.1 shows some of the chapters and their emphasis (Jima and Lakkaraju, 2014).

## Exploratory Research and Analysis

Classic experimental work in science uses a laboratory allowing control of variables with experiments holding most variables constant while systematically varying those under study. Some social-behavioral research has benefited from such laboratories (e.g., in psychological experiments, including those of the heuristics-and-biases school that originated with Daniel Kahneman and Amos Tversky). Other research has used randomized control trials (RCT), which are often thought to be the gold standard for statistical studies. Still other research has done its best to extract relationships from history and other poorly controlled data. All such methods have been exhaustively described elsewhere and need no review here.

What we do wish to highlight is a different approach, one that applies primarily to computational experimentation. This is the approach of exploratory analysis (also called exploratory modeling).

In a sense, exploratory analysis is common in computational social science, if what is meant is running large numbers of cases and seeing what can be observed. What is less common, so far, is a kind of theory-informed experimentation in which data analysis looks for patterns suggested by theory or fragments thereof, or in which machine search is used to discover patterns that may then be the basis of inferring meaningful causal relationships. Such exploratory analysis has been conducted for roughly twenty years with respect to climate change. We are also seeing exploratory computational experiments to understand epidemiological aspects of potential epidemics, sometimes as a function of vaccination efforts (Dorratoltaj et al., 2017). That work was also used to suggest a variety of practical adaptive strategies.

Some applications have been attempted in more social-behavioral settings, such as research by RAND and Lawrence Livermore National Laboratory on trader behaviors in the security industry (Dreyer et al., 2016), and in the analysis of data from massively multiplayer online games (Jima and Lakkaraju, 2014). Other applications of agent-based modeling in electric-power networks are connecting phenomena at different scales, something of considerable interest to economists as well as regulators (Tesfatsion, 2018).

A promising and important method referred to as summarization has been demonstrated with large multiagent simulations (Parikh et al., 2016). Such methods will be crucial in making sense of exploratory research with computational methods.

# Modernizing Model-Based Decision Aiding

## The Decision-Aiding Aspect of the Challenge

In describing our overall approach in Chapter 3, we identified analysis and decision aiding as a distinct topic, as suggested also in an earlier workshop that noted the importance of seeing SB models and modeling through different lenses (see also Figure 1.1, which is adapted from McNamara et al., 2011). Our study was unable to address related issues in depth, and they were not discussed in the study's workshops, but we deemed it important that the report comment on the matter, albeit tersely.

Great strides have been made over the last twenty-five years related to model-based analysis for complex problems, and some of the corresponding lessons need to be assimilated in conceiving and nurturing research on social-behavioral modeling. These lessons have implications for the building of models and their testing (verification, validation, and accreditation), design and conduct of analysis, and communication of insights to decisionmakers. We focus here exclusively on progress in dealing with uncertainty. The importance of doing so was mentioned earlier in Chapter 5 in the section "Dealing Routinely with Uncertainty," but we elaborate here. As before, we focus on the problem of deep uncertainty.

## Deep Uncertainty

Repeating the definition from Chapter 5:

> Deep uncertainty is the "condition in which analysts do not know
> or the parties to a decision cannot agree upon (1) the appropriate
> models to describe interactions among a system's variables, (2) the
> probability distributions to represent uncertainty about key par-
> ameters in the models, and/or (3) how to value the desirability of
> alternative outcomes." (Lempert et al., 2003)

The problems of deep uncertainty are not unique to the social-
behavioral realm. In DoD's planning of future military force structures, "scenario space methods" were developed to encourage looking
for force capabilities that are "flexible, adaptive, and robust" (FARness)
so that in actual crises and conflicts (actual scenarios) the capabilities
will prove apt, despite the actual scenarios departing markedly from
expectations.[1] In the study of climate-change effects, water-resource
planning, and other social problems, similar methods have come to be
called methods for "robust decisionmaking" (RDM).[2] A new and vibrant
international organization, the Society for Decision Making Under Deep
Uncertainty (DMDU), now exists (www.deepuncertainty.org) and in
November 2017 held its fifth annual meeting at Oxford University.
The name of the society is telling. The term "Decision Making" conveys a core intent: The society and its members' research is not just
about modeling, but about informing policy-level decisions at various
levels (city, state, nation, and globe).

Such work involves a shift of analytic paradigm: Instead of attempting
to optimize some outcome (subject to many dubious assumptions), the

---

[1]  See a review of RAND work on uncertainty analysis, primarily in the national security
domain (Davis, 2012), which includes pointers to literature from the early 1980s onward.

[2]  See especially Lempert et al., 2003. See also www.rand.org/topics/robust-decision-making
.html. In Europe, a center of vigorous research has been Delft University of Technology in
finding "dynamic adaptive policy pathways" for crafting robust strategies (Haasnoot et al.,
2013). Our discussion here also draws on informal presentations by Jan Kwakkel and Robert
Lempert at the November 2017 meeting of the Society for Decision Making Under Deep
Uncertainty (DMDU).

preferred strategy is one that will do "adequately" across the range of reasonable assumptions that constitute deep uncertainty. That is, one seeks strategies that are flexible, adaptive, and robust (i.e., that will accommodate changes in an objective or goal, that will accommodate unexpected circumstances, and that will deal adequately with initial shocks). Leaders in the society come from the United States, United Kingdom, Netherlands, New Zealand, and quite a number of other countries, and from organizations such as laboratories and research houses (e.g., RAND) and universities, but also the World Bank and other government offices.

## Principles and Lessons Learned

Various authors contributing to modern knowledge of how to conduct and communicate analysis have their own preferred phrases and lists, but some principles are worth expressing:[3]

- Exploratory analysis should be the core of work in supporting evaluation of possible strategies. Exploration should consider both parametric and structural uncertainties (i.e., uncertainties in the values of model variables and the models themselves). Exploration should be as comprehensive as possible, not restricted to traditional one-variable-at-a-time sensitivity analysis while holding most model inputs constant.
- So-called best-estimate predictions are of little interest given deep uncertainties. Optimizing strategy based on best-estimate predictions is often seriously counterproductive. The goal should be to find strategies that are "flexible, adaptive, and robust"—i.e., to support "robust decisionmaking."
- Strategies should be conceived from the outset so as to be adaptive over time as the actual future unfolds.

---

[3] What follows draws on a number of sources, including the senior author's work in defense applications (see Davis, 2014 and references therein), the work of RAND colleagues associated with robust decisionmaking (RDM) methods (Lempert et al., 2003) and www.rand.org/topics /robust-decision-making.html, and European researchers and analysts, notably Marjolijn Haasnoot and Jan Kwakkel (Haasnoot et al., 2013) and Erik Pruyt (Pruyt and Islam, 2015).

**Table 7.1**

**Shifts of Approach**

| From | To | Comment |
|---|---|---|
| Predict future. | Explore and understand possible futures (e.g., with well-chosen scenario sets). | Predicting is often a counterproductive goal. |
| Act on prediction (optimize for it). | Seek flexible, adaptive, and robust strategies. | Seek hedged strategy that will work adequately across as much of uncertainty space as is feasible and affordable. |
| See strategy as once and for all. | Expect and plan for appropriate adaptations. | This should include illustrating "adaptive pathways" with both continuous and discrete changes. |
| Hand analysis over the transom to inform decisionmakers. | Work with decisionmakers in interactive settings that help them learn and enrich their intuition. | This can include interactive simulations, human exercises, and an analogue to "flight simulators." |
| Expect decisionmakers to believe model results. | Expect decisionmakers to learn sensibly from modeling and interactions with models, but to be appropriately skeptical about any predictions. | Good top-level decisionmakers have typically used analysis this way. Mid-level managers often claim to the contrary that predictions are what they need. |

- In many (if not most) cases, the purpose of decision support and decision aiding should be to *facilitate learning* about a problem and courses of action, rather than as something identifying the allegedly "right" decision.

Table 7.1 summarizes these principles by drawing contrasts.

## Implications for Analysis Outputs and Communication

Such work involves a different kind of analytic output: Instead of asking a model for what will happen if . . . , or asking the model to identify the optimum strategy, we want to see how outcomes will vary

**Figure 7.1**
**Outputs of Analysis: Region Plots Indicating When a Given Strategy Will Succeed or Fail**

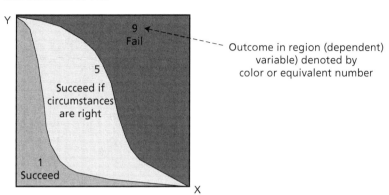

X, Y: independent variable (inputs)
Mappings: 1, 5, 9 to green (very good), yellow (marginal), and red (very bad)
RAND *RR2208-7.1*

as assumptions are changed. That is, the outputs needed are more like "region plots" or "trade-off plots." Figure 7.1 is an example. In this display, outcome is represented by color (or the equivalent number) rather than position on the y axis. The x and y axes represent the most important independent variables. The chart indicates that the strategy being evaluated will fail if the point (x, y) is anywhere in the red area (9), succeed in the green area (1), and be impossible to predict in the yellow area (5), where results would depend on all the details and perhaps random effects.

Figure 7.1 would be useful for a simple problem, but what if the number of independent variables is larger? Visualization is a problem.

Figure 7.2 shows an analysis indicating outcome as a function of five uncertain variables X, Y, Z, Q, and R. Looking at the bottom right, for example, the region in which X is very high and Y is very low, one sees that results are very bad unless Z is very high (9). Results in this corner do not depend on R or Q. Similarly, in the top left corner, results are very good independent of the variables R, Z, and Q. Thus, a strategy with very low value of X and very high value of Y is robustly good. By having four charts such as Figure 7.2 on each of two pages, one can show

# Figure 7.2
## Results as a Function of Five Variables

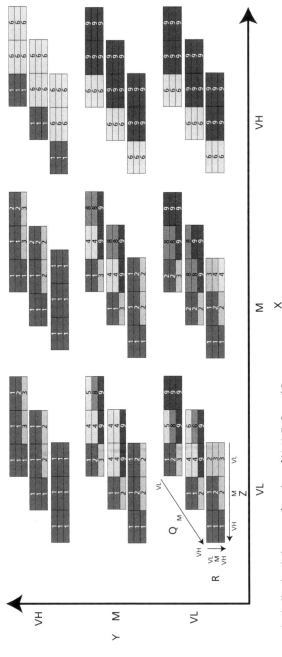

Results (cell values) shown as function of X, Y, Z, Q, and R
Notation:
VH: Very high, green, 1
H:  High, light green, 3
M:  Medium, yellow, 5
L:  Low, orange, 7
VL: Very low, red, 9
A VH as a result means very good prospects for success or for a favorable system behavior.

results of exploring over eight variables. Analogous information-dense summaries can be constructed with complex tables. In either case, the result is to allow visualization of analysis over a significantly multi-dimensional space.

Fortunately, a considerable literature of "visual analytics" now exists, as well as powerful tools such as *Tableau* (see www.tableau.com for an instructive overview). Several chapters of a MITRE book discuss visu-alization methods in some detail (Egeth et al., 2014). Visual methods play prominently in the work of those in the DMDU. See particularly related work on robust decisionmaking from RAND (www.rand. org/topics/robust-decision-making.html) and the Technical Univer-sity of Delft in the Netherlands.

When one is dealing with a sizable number of independent vari-ables, it is also possible to use modern data-mining methods so that the computer searches to find patterns indicating what combinations of independent variables drive results in portions of the n-dimensional space with substantially different outcomes. A set of methods that has proved powerful is referred to as "scenario discovery" by RAND col-leagues (Lempert et al., 2006). It uses the Patient Rule Induction Method (PRIM) data-mining algorithm developed by Jerome Friedman and Nicholas Fisher at Stanford (Friedman and Fisher, 1999).

In any case, the admonition we offer here is that it is not enough to acknowledge that uncertainties exist (but then ignore them). Instead:

- Model-based analysis should *routinely* use the methods of explor-atory analysis and *routinely* report consequences of both structural and parametric uncertainty.
- In planning contexts, such analysis should *routinely* identify strat-egies that hedge well against uncertainties—i.e., applying what has been called the FARness principle and encouraging RDM.[4]

---

[4]   See Davis, 2014, for discussion in the context of higher-level defense planning. This report also recommends a version of the admonitions here as a new ethic for analysts, one going well beyond the principle that analysts should identify the assumptions on which their analysis depends.

The implications are profound for the SBML. They mean identifying the plausible range of alternative model structures, the plausible ranges of input data, and finding ways to conduct the corresponding multidimensional analysis—not as an afterthought, but routinely.

# CHAPTER EIGHT

# Methods and Technology

This chapter is short because the syntax of most items is simply *"How in the future can we do better at . . . ?"* This question refers to the challenges acknowledged earlier. With this said, we add some discussion in what follows.

## Capacity for Multidimensional Uncertainty Analysis

Everyone favors being able to do uncertainty analysis, but no current consensus exists on how to do it, why it is not easy, and why new tools are needed. An impediment is familiarity with normal sensitivity analysis, something students learn in first-year calculus if not earlier. Sensitivity analysis is possible with more or less any model. A model is like a function F(x, y, z). One can ask how F changes if x is changed from $X_1$ to $X_2$. It is also easy to draw a chart showing F versus x with y and z held constant. So where is the problem? The problems are that (1) the methods of simple sensitivity analysis do not scale well to multiple dimensions; (2) many variables may be statistically correlated even if they are mathematically independent; (3) no useful base cases may exist around which to do minor excursions; (4) behavior of the system may change dramatically only for certain *combinations* of multiple variables, as when a system becomes unstable; (4) the usual programming languages and modeling platforms do not make multidimensional uncertainty analysis easy; and (5) modeling platforms for which it is easy are not well suited to some kinds of modeling and data analysis.[1] Nonetheless, much is known about exploratory analysis under deep uncertainty.[2]

We should also note again at this point that exploratory analysis should consider uncertainties in model structure, not just the values of its parameters. This poses additional problems for modeling platforms if they are to support uncertainty analysis broadly. Dealing with model uncertainty is a long-standing problem, but much can be done, as illustrated in recent work on heterogeneous information fusion (Davis et al., 2016).

Visualization of multidimensional uncertainty has also been studied, as in conveying complex spatial information with animation (Ehlschlaeger et al., 1997) or in representing multiple statistics (Ehlschlaeger, 2002).

## Variable-Structure Simulation and Emergence

Several of the major concerns that social scientists have with current-day simulation modeling are that the models treat as inputs important features of phenomena that are emergent in important real settings. This includes what agents exist and are important, what relationships exist among them, what "ideas" (e.g., memes) become the object of attention and social momentum, and even what value structures are at work.

If modeling is to do better on such matters, it must address an old topic that has been mentioned for decades—what is sometimes called

---

[1]    As an example, the *Analytica* platform is excellent for exploratory analysis (Davis et al., 2016), but is not suitable for agent-based or discrete-event modeling. *Vensim and Stella* are specialized for system dynamics, but are not well suited to multidimensional uncertainty analysis and are again not suitable for agent-based modeling. Some other platforms have broader capabilities but are currently quite expensive. We are not aware of an up-to-date review on such matters.

[2]    See Chapter 5 ("Toward Multivariate Causal Models") and related research being done at Delft University (Pruyt and Kwakkel, 2014; Pruyt and Islam, 2015), but the methods and tools are still relatively young and sometimes require a degree of virtuosity with programming and data-handling tools. Visualizations and other expressions of output are not yet adequate. We observe that, despite initial promises about doing uncertainty analysis, it is common for projects to end up with only minimal levels because the programming language and/or the programs they have written are unsuitable. What *might* have been built in from the start is very difficult to build in as an afterthought.

variable-structure simulation. Further, new thinking and tools will be needed to manage the resulting capabilities once they exist.

How best to go about such challenges is unclear. Much can be done in some cases by building in all necessary structure at the outset and allowing elements of the structure to be turned on or off as the system evolves, or for groupings to come and go. This approach occurs in dynamic network analysis (Breiger et al., 2003; Carley, 2006). It was also used in 1980s-era "analytic war gaming" with alternative aggregate-level agents representing the top leadership of the Soviet Union and United States, each of which also had alternative war plans. As the simulation proceeded, war plans could be changed and the analyst could decree a change of leadership mindset (i.e., the analyst could say, "Suppose that a coup occurs and the Red agent changes character. What then?").[3]

Levent Yilmaz and Tuncer Ören have written on related matters, sometimes using the terminology of self-aware simulations (Yilmaz, 2006a; Yilmaz and Ören, 2009). Sometimes it is referred to as allowing "reflection" in simulations (Uhrmacher et al., 2002). Some cross-platform work has been reported (Mehlhase, 2014).

## Knowledge Management and Heterogeneous Information Fusion

A broad concern is that while a great deal of knowledge about social-behavioral matters exists, even a great deal of knowledge specifically relevant to social-behavioral modeling, it exists in many different communities and is expressed in different specialized terminology and forms (e.g., essays, maps, survey data, data from laboratory experiments, and computer models of varied types, in different languages). We have mentioned some of this earlier, when acknowledging sharp differences between, say, the narratives of anthropologists and economists, but the overall challenge is bigger and multifaceted. It is becoming even bigger in the Internet of Everything (IoE) era. We are in the

---

[3]   See Davis, 1989, and documents cited therein.

early stages of learning how to manage the knowledge effectively and how to combine the many forms of information. We mention only two examples of prior work here, so as to whet the appetites of readers.

A survey paper on intrusion detection addresses many of the more generic issues (Zeuch et al., 2015). It describes relevant modern technologies and expresses optimism: "Overall, both cyber threat analysis and cyber intelligence could be enhanced by correlating security events across many diverse heterogeneous sources" (p. 1). Although the paper is more about empirical data than theory or modeling, much in the paper should apply to the challenges of social-behavioral modeling.

Another study was a basic research effort on how to fuse heterogeneous information ranging from human-source accounts to digital records when some of that information may be ambiguous, contradictory, or even the result of deliberate deception (Davis et al., 2016). The purpose of the research was improving the ability both to detect individuals who pose a terrorist threat and to exonerate those falsely accused. The authors envisioned a human-in-the-loop approach, rather than the more commonly studied automated methods. They saw it as essential to represent subjective judgments, including bimodal probabilistic judgments, and to then anticipate senior human analysts applying a mix of art and science to sharpen assessments. They saw intermediate output for an individual along these lines:

> This individual is *probably* not a threat, but there is a distinct probability that he is and we lack the information to know that. We need information on his capabilities and accesses as a priority. It is also possible that the adverse information on him is misleading, since it is all based on two sources of data that, upon reflection, are correlated and could be the result of false accusations. Thus, we need further information about the accuser.

The platform used built-in capability for uncertainty analysis about both model structure and parameter values. Heterogeneous fusion was accomplished with several competing algorithms (e.g., a quasi-Bayesian method and an entropy maximizing method), and the data used for each was treated as uncertain. If results agreed, analysis could stop; if they disagreed, then human analysts would need to go deeper, sometimes going back to original data to better assess which methods were more credible in the specific case. The authors also considered briefly how alternative narratives could be brought to bear (essentially as meta-level models causing human analysts to interpret data differently).

## Composability

The challenges of model composability were discussed in Chapter 2. Although progress has been made as noted in earlier citations and a recent review from a computer science perspective (Levis, 2016), the deeper issues are resistant to mathematical or technological breakthroughs. Researchers have to understand the models to be composed, the assumptions that underlie them, the contexts (regions of their state spaces) in which they will be exercised, and the purpose of the composition. The problems are different in degree from those in the well-developed literature on component-based software engineering and different in type from those discussed in some other engineering-oriented papers (Szyperski, 2002). This said, the problem may be "impossible in principle but more tractable in practice." In a given study, researchers can address the issues, as some have done in multimodeling experiments in recent years that addressed complex political, military, and economic interactions in simulated intervention operations (Lofdahl, 2010) and connecting agent-based network models and a system-dynamic-style model (Carley, 2012; Levis et al., 2010). It seems that great advances could be made with a combination of (1) a concept of best practices, (2) methods that organize thinking about composition, (3) modular development with better documentation and comprehensibility, and (4) technology that facilitates following the best practices, including systematic testing across the relevant state space and documenting as much as possible assumptions that otherwise would merely be in the head of the modeler/programmer.

Among the considerations in improving the ability to compose models as needed for a particular effort will be the need to develop accessible and community-vetted libraries of lower-level modules. This suggestion is rather unexceptionable given the great value that modelers worldwide see in libraries for algorithms and other matters. For the domain of interest in this paper, however, the libraries should have additional characteristics:

- The "taxonomy" of modules should make sense from a scientific perspective.
- The modules should be comprehensible, designed for uncertainty analysis, and peer-reviewed (not for being "definitive," but rather for doing well what they do).
- Competitive versions of the same modules are needed to represent alternative theories, alternative perspectives, and alternative techniques.
- Ideally, the "controlled" version of a given module should be expressed either in a language-independent manner (e.g., logic, mathematics, pseudocode) or in a very high-level language that makes comprehending theory easily possible.

As discussed in earlier sections, much can and should be done to improve the comprehensibility of models, which will in turn enable peer review and debate among scientists who need not be good programmers. Related improvements can also be made in reproducibility and shareability. Many good ideas on the matter have been suggested, but much remains to be done.[4]

## Theory-Informed Empirical and Computational Experimentation

We have discussed the need for more theory-informed experimentation (see Chapter 6, "Exploratory Research and Analysis"), but how to do so is a matter very much in its infancy. The value of the

---

[4]  Volker Grimm and associates have suggested a protocol for documenting agent-based models. This is the Overview, Design concept, Details (ODD) protocol. It seems to have broad applicability (Grimm et al., 2010).

computational experimentation was anticipated well by Joshua Epstein some years ago:

> The agent-based computational model is a new tool for empirical research. It offers a natural environment for the study of connectionist phenomena in social science. Agent-based modeling provides a powerful way to address certain enduring—and especially interdisciplinary—questions. It allows one to subject certain core theories—such as neoclassical microeconomics—to important types of stress (e.g., the effect of evolving preferences). It permits one to study how rules of individual behavior give rise—or "map up"—to macroscopic regularities and organizations. In turn, one can employ laboratory behavioral research findings to select among competing agent-based ("bottom up") models. The agent-based approach may well have the important effect of decoupling individual rationality from macroscopic equilibrium and of separating decision science from social science more generally. Agent-based modeling offers powerful new forms of hybrid theoretical-computational work; these are particularly relevant to the study of non-equilibrium systems. (Epstein, 1999)

In subsequent years, Epstein has pursued this agenda in ways that do indeed cross disciplines and provide vision of how to construct more coherent theory, as suggested in his Agent Zero work (Epstein, 2014). Agent Zero, although deliberately simple, is endowed with distinct emotional/affective, cognitive/deliberative, and social modules. Further, it is informed by several disciplines, including modern neuroscience.

Many pitfalls exist. In particular, as described by Robert Axtell and colleagues, the usefulness of the exploratory computation possible with agent-based models depends on the reasonableness of the elementary logic written into the agents. Axtell laments the state of affairs in that regard and yearns for better insights from the social-behavioral scientists. What is needed are theory-informed "specifications" that can be used to define agent characteristics in ABM work.

Given results of computational experiments, how might they be analyzed and displayed for better comprehension? And how might that be theory informed? Based on work with which we are more or less familiar, we see the need for a combination of analytic artistry and systematic method. In our own work, which has relied more on visual search, multiresolution theory and modeling has made it possible to anticipate patterns and then verify or falsify them with visual search of outcome data (Davis et al., 2007). In colleagues' work on applications of robust decisionmaking (RDM), machine methods have proved powerful in finding meaningful patterns in a process that the authors call scenario discovery (Groves and Lempert, 2007; Popper et al., 2010). Success, however, depends in part on giving the machine theory-informed hints about the variables to use in looking for patterns. Those hints can be much better with even a qualitatively expressed multiresolution theory.

## Interactivity, Gaming, and Related Visualization

Many advances have occurred in recent years with respect to interactivity in simulations and using human gaming (or other human exercises) for serious exploration and problem solving. Visualization is an important element of most such work.[5]

## Other

Among the many other issues, we mention without elaboration:

1. How do we make the best use of modern data sources, which are sometimes massive, sometimes sparse, and often riddled with subtle correlations?
2. How do we infer likely causal relations from only partially controlled observational data?

---

[5] Examples are Michael Zyda's work on serious games (Zyda, 2007); William Rouse's work using modeling and simulation to inform and work directly with leadership of various organizations (Rouse and Boff, 2005), including health care organizations (Rouse, 2015); and "explorable explanations" (Hart and Case, undated), such as animated ways to study Thomas Schelling's model of how segregation may occur due to on-the-margin preferences (Schelling, 1971).

3.  What should output look like—along the way during research and, later, when informing decisionmakers or the public? How can communication be improved when dealing with multidimensional issues, balancing depth and breadth, and using cognitively effective mechanisms? Solutions will presumably include depictions of outcome metrics in n-dimensional space, but comprehensible versions are as difficult to design as, say, "intuitive" interfaces for complex personal digital devices.[6]

---

[6]  An interesting effort of this type has involved exploratory computational experimentation on cyberwar issues, intended to be useful to military cyberwarriors (Dobson and Carley, 2017). Another effort uses qualitative modeling to inform discussion and displays for human war games and other exercises (Davis, 2017).

# CHAPTER NINE

# Infrastructure, Culture, and Governance

To complete our walk through the ecostructure indicated in Figure 1.2, this chapter touches on issues of infrastructure, culture, and governance. These topics deal less with research than with management, but we see it as crucial for the overall DARPA effort to do its part in achieving major shifts:

1.  Change the cultural and intellectual mindset from one that sees model-based analysis in terms of narrow point predictions and optimization (akin to engineering) and move toward analysis of wicked problems and development of robust strategies. Change the nature of demands for analysis and its products accordingly.
2.  Consistent with this change, encourage a mindset of adaptive strategy, which requires monitoring and adaptation, rather than a single decision and implementation.
3.  Encourage a mindset that sees "human terrain" as complex, dynamic, and heterogeneous, rather than as something to be characterized definitively in databases.

Another whole class of issues involves the ethics of ensuring privacy and respect for human rights.

## Infrastructure

The relevant elements of infrastructure include (1) vigorous academic and private-world research programs in numerous institutions in the

United States and other countries, (2) related funding, and (3) mechanisms for interaction. It includes having laws, regulations, funding strategies, and relationships that encourage the right balances among, for example, openness, sharing, and protection of intellectual property.

## Cultural Mindsets

Mismatches currently exist—among both recipients of research and the researchers themselves—between what is sought and what *should* be sought in describing knowledge and informing reasoned decision-making. Mindset changes are needed, especially in the domain of social-behavioral issues. Table 9.1 summarizes them.

These changes in mindset would be consistent with a large body of modern research in the decision sciences and applications to planning problems.

**Table 9.1**
**Cultural Mindset Changes**

| From | To |
| --- | --- |
| Seeking narrow point predictions and optimization (akin to engineering) | Seeking analysis of wicked problems and development of robust strategies |
| Seeking a simple once-and-for-all strategy | Seeking explicitly adaptive strategies that require routine monitoring and adjustment |
| Seeking "human terrain" with solid, fixed data | Seeing the "terrain" as complex, heterogeneous, and dynamic—in structure, not just attribute values |
| Predicting and acting | Exploring and proceeding with adaptation expected |
| Using unvalidated models or using generically validated models to inform particular important decisions | Deemphasizing "generic" validation and elevating the importance of analysis-specific validation |
| Receiving and acting on model-generated answers | Interacting with models to understand systems and phenomena, including relationships, possibilities, and potential adaptations |

## Governance and Ethics, Privacy, and Civil Liberties

### Results from a Workshop on Ethics and Privacy

Another whole class of issues involves the ethics of ensuring privacy and respect for civil liberties. It is to be expected that many elements of research will involve data collection and data analysis, some of which could—without strong, well-conceived protections—cause difficulties and, in some instances, violate the intentions of law. DARPA intends to maintain and help establish the highest standards on such matters, but to do so will require continued analysis and innovation, and perhaps promulgation of suitable laws. This was the subject of a previous workshop. The summary from that workshop (Balebako et al., 2017) stated that:

> The RAND study team identified six important topics to consider for reducing problems related to privacy and harms caused by misuse of personal data, ranging from how individuals are notified of data use, to how to deter harms arising from data use. The topics were how to:
> - Ensure *meaningful* user notice and choice.
> - Provide usable and accurate access control.
> - Anonymize data.
> - Validate and audit data algorithms to avoid inadvertent harms.
> - Challenge and redress data harms.
> - Deter abuse.
>
> Looking across these six issues, we had three main observations:
>
> Developing solutions to prevent harms caused by misuse of personal data is difficult, complicated, and beset by tensions (no simple divide exists between "good guys" and "bad guys").
>
> The challenges of and potential solutions to data harms are interrelated. For example, providing mechanisms for redress are intertwined with increasing transparency about how data are used.
>
> Single-approach solutions are unlikely to be effective. Decisionmakers should adopt a portfolio approach that looks for *mixes* of incentives, education, market solutions, and related technologies, government regulations, and standards. The either-or fallacy should be avoided: It is evident that, in most of the problem areas, a mixed approach is *necessary* for success.

The report goes on to identify priority topics for attention and action.

**More General Ethical Reasons for Caution**

Much more research is needed to better understand the scope of challenges involving ethics, privacy, civil liberties, and the sometimes-insidious ways that increased but imperfect knowledge (and related modeling) can be used in counterproductive and sometimes terrible ways. As one example, earlier periods in the study of anthropology promoted ideas that we now recognize as outrageously racist as well as scientifically wrong (Konner, 2003). As a modern example, social science empirical research has generated statistical models that predict the probability that a criminal defendant will commit further crimes, something used by courts in deciding on incarceration. Even if the software and underlying data were accurate and precise (which is unlikely), moral and ethical issues loom large when applying the aggregate-level model to individuals. The underlying problems are deep: For example, optimizing the model to ensure comparable predictions of future crime for people of different races leads to unfairness of outcomes (with error rates being greater for one race than another).[1] Learning how to construct algorithms with fairer outcomes is an important research topic, not only in criminal justice but in many applications of social science that could be supported by social-behavioral models.[2]

---

[1]  We thank Dr. Laura McNamara, one of the reviewers of our draft report, for this example. A related technical paper discusses a fairness criterion for supervised-learning applications (Hardt et al., 2017). A news article describes the larger policy debate and its dilemmas (Angwin and Larson, 2017).

[2]  See also a book that excoriates bad use of modeling that the authors believe has seriously misinformed environmental policies (Pilkey and Pilkey-Jarvis, 2007). The primary culprits are said to be quantitative modelers who have an almost religiously fanatic outlook on the veracity of their models. In contrast, they observe, qualitative models are assessed much more positively.

## Final Comments

This report has described what we see as priority challenges for social and behavioral modeling. Some of the obstacles to progress reflect inherent challenges: Social systems are complex adaptive systems; they often pose "wicked problems"; and even the structure of social systems shows emergent behavior. Other obstacles reflect disciplinary norms and practices, mindsets, and very difficult scientific and methodological challenges.

We recommend an overall strategy that is more problem focused than usual work so as to force interdisciplinary efforts and encourage breakthroughs. Identifying a small number of national challenges and then confronting each of them in separate strands of work could prove effective. This could be accomplished with what we have called virtual social-behavioral modeling laboratories that would cross disciplinary and methodological boundaries as necessary to address the concrete problems. Doing so might encourage a new style of knowledge building.

For each national challenge problem, we discussed challenges in six groups:

1. Improving the research cycle by tightening links among theory, modeling, and experimentation.
2. Seeking more unifying and coherent theories while retaining alternative perspectives and confronting multidimensional uncertainty from the outset.
3. Invigorating experimentation with modern data sources that are increasingly informed by theory-observation iteration.
4. Modernizing ways to use social-behavioral models for analysis to aid decisionmaking, in particular by drawing on lessons learned from other domains about using models to assist planning under deep uncertainty.
5. Challenging theorists and technologists to provide related methods and tools, since existing ones are inadequate and often counterproductive.
6. Nurturing the rest of the ecology (notably infrastructure, governance, and culture) needed for overall effectiveness, and doing

so in a way that adheres to the highest standards with regard to ethics, privacy, and responsible use of model-based analysis to inform policy decisions that may have profound effects.

The report's ten-page summary mirrors the structure of the full report but can be read as a stand-alone.

# Social and Behavioral Modeling Laboratories

## Introduction

Chapter 3 of the main text sketched the concept of social and behavioral modeling laboratories (SBMLs) as a mechanism for advancing knowledge. This appendix describes in greater detail an illustrative design for an SBML approach. Although merely illustrative, it attempts to address the multiple facets of such an approach concretely, thereby illuminating what would be involved.

SBMLs would be a way to produce meaningful and lasting progress and of gaining insight into the ways in which social media and other communication media interact with society. The concept is *not* one of having some centralized, official, single simulation in a government computer somewhere, but rather creating an improved distributed ecology to facilitate cross- and interdisciplinary work and to develop an evolving collection of accepted, broadly applicable, modular components and related pieces of research to formalize, advance, and combine models from across the social sciences. The research would occur in academia, national laboratories, and other private and commercial research organizations. We anticipate different SBMLs for different challenge problems.

The SBMLs would include distributed platforms for researchers to use in running experiments "in silico" and comparing with empirical information and theory. This could help understand, interpret, and provisionally predict (with uncertainties) social outcomes that could in turn be used to guide investment, assess strategy, and formulate interventions. SBMLs would also allow for human gaming and hybrid simulations in which people and models would be used interchangeably.

The SBMLs would provide a way for social science ideas to be formalized, tested, debated, competed, and to evolve. In other words, they would enable better and more rigorous advancement of the science, not just applications of the science.

## A Social-Behavioral Modeling Laboratory (SBML)

If an SBML is to operate as a decentralized modeling environment, it will depend on incentives and governance to maintain focus and quality. This section outlines practical principles for setting and maintaining this environment.

The National Research Council (Zacharias et al., 2008, pp. 356–369) made recommendations for military-sponsored modeling research that provide a solid foundation for the governance of an SBML. It identified both problem categories and areas for research (see this report's Table 1.2 for the main themes from the 2008 NRC report).

The NRC also laid out a high-level roadmap for recommended research. This roadmap is based on the idea of "use-driven research" as described by Donald Stokes in a book that challenged Vannevar Bush's stark contrast in 1945 between basic and applied research. Stokes drew in part on Louis Pasteur's work for inspiration: Pasteur's work was *both* a quest for fundamental understanding *and* very useful (Stokes, 1997). Use-driven research strikes a balance between basic and applied research— seeking answers to practical problems while at the same time continually coming back to fundamental questions of why some methods work and others do not.

This process (and the strategy we suggest in Chapter 2) would be driven by a version of use-driven work, one in which "challenge problems" guide each funding and development cycle. The chronology over a period of time might be as in Table A.1. The challenge problems would guide specification of the uses to which models would be put and the criteria for judging their success. At the end of a given funding cycle, a model's built-in response to the challenge would be evaluated to gauge its utility in addressing the question. This might result in further model development, new modeling tools, new social science or modeling theory, and refinement, expansion, and clarification of the challenge question for use in further funding cycles. After a funding cycle has been formally evaluated, a new funding cycle would address previous shortcomings.

The challenge-problem approach is well suited to the development of SBMLs. Early challenge problems would provide contexts for developing behavioral frameworks and demonstrating modular approaches within these frameworks. Funding calls would make this criterion explicit, and proposals would be evaluated as much for their ability to demonstrate understanding of, and commitment to, the development of workable frameworks as they would be for substantive expertise and ability to make progress on the social science problem itself.

The NRC further recommended that the funding agency hold annual conferences for funded researchers geared toward learning about the challenge problem and becoming familiar with data sets that might be relevant to the problem. After the first year, these conferences would be coupled with validation workshops with both modelers and representative users (perhaps the same people) who would be in a position

Table A.1
**Possible Chronology of Events in the History of a Social-Behavioral Modeling Laboratory**

| Year One | Subsequent Years | All Years |
|---|---|---|
| Statement of challenge problem | Enriched challenge statement | Workshops and conferences for: |
| Call for systematic approaches to the challenge problem producing framework, modules, system platform, and prototype application | Call for systematic approaches encouraging use or extension of existing frameworks and modules | Discussion Dissemination Validation Reflection Scientific advisory board Comparison and debate of specific frameworks and modules |
| Results, review, conclusions | Calls for modules implementing specific social science theories for existing frameworks | |
| | Calls for models that make use of existing frameworks and modules (if mature, may be handed off to other agencies) | |

to evaluate how useful the developed models are, given their intended purpose. Feedback would help formulate the challenge problems and funding priorities for the next annual cycle.

## Implementing the Use-Driven Cycle

While the 2008 NRC report describes the use-driven research cycle at a high level, the details of its implementation would be critical to success. The process requires leadership that would digest the results of funded research along with general progress in the field, generate new challenge questions, and maintain high quality. This is likely to require experienced DARPA staff and scientific advisory boards. The advisory boards might function much like the program committee of a scientific conference. A subset of the board would provide peer review on each project well before the validation workshop so that researchers would have time to address comments. This would ensure that the work presented at the workshop had face validity coming in, thus freeing the workshop participants to focus on deeper issues relating to fitness for purpose, conceptual scope, etc.

Soon after the validation workshop, the advisory committee would meet with DARPA staff to digest the presented work, identify progress made in the current cycle, point out shortcomings and challenges that the work has brought to light, suggest new areas of inquiry that have emerged, and develop a candidate set of challenge problems for the next cycle. This process would likely benefit from seeding by DARPA staff, who might begin the meeting with thoughts on these items based both on the pre-workshop review and the presentations and discussions of the workshop itself.

After this advisory committee meeting, DARPA staff would transform the material from the workshop into a challenge problem and set of funding priorities for the next cycle. These would be embedded within specific funding calls that would be put out as soon after the validation workshop as is practical.

Given the lead time for review before the workshop, and the time it would take to digest workshop proceedings and generate new funding calls, a one-year cycle would not be workable. Instead, funding should be granted over various time frames ranging from one to three years, depending on the type of call. We anticipate three general types of call: Frameworks, Applied Models, and Module Development. We also anticipate the need to address explicitly issues of process, timeliness, and the building of scientific and craft knowledge with the intent of achieving the kind of vibrant, productive "epistemic culture" that partly motivates our concept of SBMLs.

## Illustrative Challenge Problems

Challenge problems should be specific enough to focus research yet broad enough to allow for strongly interdisciplinary work. Preferably, they should focus on issues that present current and real challenges to policymakers, where there is reason to believe that computer-driven modeling will be useful and where progress to date has not been adequate enough to drive solid decisionmaking.

Examples of useful challenge questions:

- What drives people to commit violent extremist acts, and how can appeals be reduced?
- Why have United States politics become so polarized and what, if anything, might be done to mitigate problems?
- What changes in the U.S. economy and social fabric may be brought about by the widespread adoption of driverless cars?
- As evidence mounts about human-induced climate change and its potentially catastrophic impacts, what kinds of changes to norms, attitudes, and governance might develop as a response?
- When international interventions are necessary in the wake of civil wars, how can they best be managed?
- How should governments prepare for managing behaviors of populations after natural disasters?
- How can federal and state governments best deal with the current opioid and obesity epidemics in the United States?

## Behavioral Frameworks

Framework calls would request the development of frameworks (modular architectures) for representing social behavior at one or a set of levels of abstraction. As discussed in the main text, it is anticipated that no single modular architecture would be able to encompass all relevant problems. However, it seems plausible that a curated set of such architectures might provide coherence without overly limiting the range of conceptual expression.[1]

Criteria for evaluating framework proposals would include the degree to which a proposed framework is extensible to cover a broad range of uses, the extent to which it facilitates modular behavioral representation, and the extent to which it can be grounded in established science (including both cognitive/behavioral science and computer science). Behavioral framework deliverables should include at least one (and likely more than one) demonstration model that makes use of the framework, demonstrates its utility, and can serve as a paradigm for future projects that use the same framework.

These calls would likely have a relatively long funding cycle—at least three years. This would allow time to do substantial work, including both social science and software engineering. It would also enable the researchers that develop a framework to collaborate with other funded researchers, working under other types of calls, who would make use of the framework in succeeding cycles.

## Module Development

Module development calls would present focused, one-year funding opportunities aimed at translating established social science into reusable modules within the behavioral frameworks outlined above. Some of the calls would be aimed not at producing fundamentally new science, but rather on the difficult task of translating accepted social science

---

[1]  One example of a nascent framework is that of "Agent Zero," as described by Joshua Epstein (Epstein, 2014).

observations and theories into functional, well-documented models that can be used by other researchers within the SBML context.

Criteria for evaluating proposals and projects would include the expertise of the project team in both the relevant social science and information technology realms, the potential breadth of applicability of the proposed module or modules, and the extent to which the proposal integrates with and makes good use of the behavioral framework it seeks to extend.

The deliverable for module development projects would include the conceptual model, a specified model, and software code representing the module; thorough documentation and linkages to published work in social science; and at least one demonstration model using the module in a manner consistent with behavioral framework of which it is a part. This demonstration model would be expected to illustrate a documented pattern from the social science literature but would not necessarily be expected to contribute to new knowledge in social science.

Module development calls would not be issued until the SBML had produced at least one workable framework—probably not earlier than year three of its existence. Modules, as envisioned here, would be extensions of an existing framework that add to its capabilities by incorporating established social science into the framework. Thus, the framework needs to exist and be reasonably well understood before such a call would make sense.

## Applied Models

Once one or more behavioral frameworks have been demonstrated and at least a handful of modules are in place, calls can be made for applied work that uses the frameworks and existing modules to address current questions in social science. These models are the ultimate aim of the SBML project, but they should rely strongly on the framework and module libraries created in response to the framework and module calls. These projects would respond directly to the current challenge question and may bring together various strands of new and existing social science research in the form of models within the simulator environment. These projects would be expected to make substantive contributions to either social science or operational capability.

Funding duration for these calls would probably not be less than two years, thereby allowing funded researchers to participate in more than one cycle of validation workshop and feedback. Sustained interaction with the SBML ecosystem would be essential to building the community of scientists and modeling practitioners to drive real progress. Applied projects would likely maintain their focus on the challenge question under which they were funded over the multiple years of their funding. This would make for a mix of challenge questions being addressed in each validation workshop, as the question would be updated or changed at the beginning of each funding cycle. The resulting limited mix of focus areas should help to sustain the generality of the simulator work program.

Criteria for evaluating proposals and projects would include not only the project's contribution to scientific understanding and operational capability, but also the extent to which the project makes use of—and extends—one or more of the behavioral frameworks. Applied models should ideally make use of some existing behavioral modules and also produce new modules that are, themselves, potentially reusable by future researchers.

## Mechanisms for Quality Control

It is expected that researchers would find ways to improve and/or extend these modules. If managed well, this would have the potential to produce steady incremental progress. If managed badly, this process could result in chaotic changes, inconsistent models, and muddled representations of theory. Improvement of existing modules should be encouraged, but all changes should be reviewed for quality and consistency with established theory.

The maintenance of a high-quality repository will require a degree of governance. Procedures should be developed for documenting all changes to existing modules. This should include the conceptual model, the specified model (if separate), as well as the implemented code itself (and code-level comments), but also an explanation for the changes and citations to relevant literature that provides the ideas underlying the changes. Changes to modules should be reviewed as part of the preparation for the annual validation workshop. If possible, the author of the original module and of the framework of which it is a part should be consulted as well. If, after this peer-review process, the changes are found to be valid and to improve on the functionality of the module, the modified module should be placed back into the system as the standard module for that aspect of social behavior.

In software development, major efforts are often made to preserve backward compatibility in the face of such changes—ensuring that any changes in functionality are limited to new method calls but do not affect existing ones (except for coding errors, which should simply be fixed). Backward compatibility may not be required in this case. Older models might continue to use the modules that they were designed with, but new models would tend to use the latest community-accepted versions.

## Repositories

Because work would be distributed among funded researchers, facilitating reuse and extension would require repositories for models and data. A repository would contain several types of items: conceptual model, specified model (if separate), code, social science data, formal metadata, and descriptions (research notes, journal articles, etc.). The repository would document the progress of the SBML project, manage model code, perform version control, and allow researchers to browse and understand frameworks, modules, and models. The repository would also be designed to facilitate discussion, allowing for the posting of comments on the various items it contains.

If well designed, the repository would be a major part of the fabric of the social and behavioral modeling community. While it is conceivable that the repository would be publicly viewable, it is more likely that it would be open only to people affiliated with the SBML project.

That said, it might be wise to provide access to a broad range of trusted researchers, whether or not they are working on an actively funded project.

Use of the frameworks, modules, and models stored in the repository might be licensed under a "copyleft" scheme resembling the GNU General Public License (GPL), with an important variation. Whereas the GPL requires that any derivative products be provided to the public free of charge under the same GPL license, the SBML license would require that all derivative products be provided back to the repository free of charge. This would encourage a range of computational social scientists to use, improve, and build the simulator codebase, as well as expose the models to more rigorous scientific scrutiny.

A given repository could make use of a number of existing tools for content management and version control. In addition to document and discussion management (which might be accomplished with a host of commercial off-the-shelf or open-source systems), the repository would need to host a code base that might involve code written in a large number of languages. This could be accomplished through the use of an open-source version control system (e.g., Git).

To remain clean and useful, a repository would require curation and maintenance. This task might be conducted by DARPA staff or be contracted out to a competent party, such as a national laboratory with continuity of relevant capability. It would be essential that the repository not become cluttered or out of date. While researcher-generated, bottom-up content would be the primary driver of the repository, it would take strong top-down management to ensure that projects are presented and documented in a consistent way. One way to encourage this would be to make the repository the primary source for deliverables on the projects. The peer reviews conducted prior to the annual validation workshops would, for example, be conducted based solely on the materials that the researcher had placed in the repository. This would encourage the development of norms and standards for documentary materials, thereby allowing clear understanding and evaluation of each piece of research that was part of the SBML environment.

# Conclusion

The SBML concept outlined here includes some inherent tensions. In a challenge-problem approach (a kind of use-driven approach), the premium is on advancing knowledge relevant to the problem and its solution. However, one purpose of an SBML would be to promote a degree of standardization and reusability. These purposes could be at odds. Balancing them would be a challenge in itself. We are influenced by the unfortunate example of campaign modeling in the Department of Defense. Great progress was made in standardization and dissemination of standard models and databases, but a consequence was major obfuscation of uncertainty and a failure to address clearly and convincingly the problems on which policymakers wanted to focus. The result, after many years, was that policymakers disestablished major elements of the campaign-modeling enterprise. This was very controversial, with good arguments on both sides, but it illustrates the dangers that can befall modeling activities when they overemphasize standardization. One of us (Davis) reviewed this matter in a congressionally mandated study (P. Davis, 2016).

If these tensions can be successfully managed, we believe that an SBML approach along the lines presented here has the potential to create a set of multiresolution, data-rich social and behavioral laboratories that promote both cooperation (through openness of code and documentation) and competition (through funding and recognition) among social scientists, and that these laboratories would offer a new and useful method for pulling together existing advances in computational social science into a rich contextual environment and making that environment available to enable further advances. We suggest that this environment should not take the form of a monolithic model of everything, or even of a closed modeling environment. Rather, we have outlined the design of a more standards-based modeling and simulation ecosystem that uses behavioral frameworks to coordinate modular components into useful models. These frameworks, and conceptual, specified, and implemented modules and models would be developed in a structured funding cycle with peer review and annual validation workshops to ensure that the work reflects accepted social science knowledge and has been done in a way that will maximize the ability of future researchers to reuse and build on past work.

# Definitions

## Official Definitions

The DoD's official definitions are (Department of Defense, 2009, pp. 9–10) as follows:

> Model. A physical, mathematical, or otherwise logical representation of a system, entity, phenomenon, or process.
>
> Simulation. A method for implementing a model over time. (Examples: a federation, distributed interactive simulation, combinations of simulations).
>
> Validation. The process of determining the degree to which a model or simulation and its associated data are an accurate representation of the real world from the perspective of the intended uses of the model.
>
> Verification. The process of determining that a model or simulation implementation and its associated data accurately represent the developer's conceptual description and specifications.

## Other Definitions

The official definition of "simulation" is confusing and only one of many across communities. A simpler definition suitable to this report is as follows:

A "simulation model" is a model that describes the behavior of a system *over time*. A simulation is the act of executing a simulation model—i.e., "running it." The mechanism for doing so is sometimes called a "simulator" (e.g., generic software for driving various simulation models).

Other confusing terms include "internal validity" and "external validity." These terms are common in some branches of science, but have numerous definitions across sources. We use them to refer to whether a specific study is done "right," with sound conclusions *given* the study's assumptions and context, and whether the conclusions generalize beyond that narrow context, respectively.

**Table B.1**
**Other Definitions**

| Term | Meaning |
|---|---|
| Abductive | A type of inference that interprets information in terms of the explanation that seems best pragmatically. |
| Explanation | In statistical analysis, a model's explanation capability refers to the fraction of the variance of data associated with the explicit terms of the regression equation; in causal analysis, a model's explanation capability is the degree to which the model gives a credible and understandable causal story with which the data is consistent. The two meanings may be at odds: A statistical model may explain the observed data very well but be regarded as having no explanatory power from the viewpoint of causal theory. |
| Exploratory analysis (EA) | Analysis based on generating model outputs over the entire n-dimensional space of the model's inputs, including model structure. |
| Exploratory modeling (EM) | Used synonymously with EA. |
| Multiresolution modeling (MRM) | Modeling that allows the user to make inputs at alternative levels of detail with acceptable degrees of consistency; may be accomplished in a single model or with a family of models. |
| Multiresolution, multiperspective modeling (MRMPM) | Modeling that includes MRM and alternative perspectives, as when model structure changes with narrative or coordinate system. |
| Robust decisionmaking (RDM) | A particular method for finding "robust strategies" that should do well across the plausible range of input assumptions. |

Internal and external validity do not correspond to verification and validation of model-based study, and the relationships between the two terminologies are probably not resolvable without major changes of definition. In the modeling, simulation, and analysis (MS&A) realm, "verification" refers to whether a computer program correctly represents the model being used (for the context of use). Using such a verified program does not imply internal validity test, however, because the model itself might be mathematically or otherwise logically wrong. Establishing internal validity, then, covers *some* of what is involved in establishing model validity. However, a statistical analysis may be regarded as internally valid even though the statistical analysis is *mis-specified*. For example, the statistical analysis might treat X, Y, and Z as independent variables, but the theory might argue that $Q = (X + Y + Z)$ is the suitable independent variable. Statistical analysis might conclude that X, Y, and Z each have modest effect, whereas—with the theory-informed specification—Q would be shown to have a moderate or large effect.

# Validation

A considerable literature exists on model verification and validation (V&V), much of it developed originally for the U.S. Department of Defense[1] but with extensive generalizations to other modeling domains.[2] We discuss only validation, supplementing material in the main text (Chapter 2, "Rethinking Model Validity"). Verification is also very important, but that is recognized and we see the challenges as technical rather than scientific or analytic.

Most of the relevant literature on validation focuses on physical systems and has a heritage in engineering (Youngblood et al., 2000; Pace, 2004). What people usually have in mind when referring to validation is establishing that predictions of a system's performance are "close enough" to measurements on the performance of a real physical system (e.g., perhaps with 10 percent for some class of experimental conditions). More careful discussions emphasize that "close enough" must be judged in a well-defined "experimental frame" that specifies all relevant variables of circumstance, including how results will be used (Zeigler, 1998; Zeigler et al., 2000).

The DoD's definitions are (Defense Modeling and Simulation Coordination Office, 2016):

- Verification: the process of determining that a model or simulation implementation and its associated data accurately

---

[1] DoD maintains a website on best practice for what DoD refers to as verification, validation, and accreditation (VV&A). See also Thacker et al., 2004.

[2] An entry to the classic literature for predictive models is an NRC study (Adams and Hidden, 2012) that deals with complex physics and engineering models. An earlier NRC study addressed environment-related models (Whipple, 2007).

represent the developer's conceptual description and specifications.

• Validation: the process of determining the degree to which a model
or simulation and its associated data are an accurate representation of the real world from the perspective of the intended uses of
the model.

• Accreditation: the official certification that a model or simulation
and its associated data are acceptable for use for a specific purpose.

Insightful discussions of validation have long appeared in the
system dynamics literature, although usually in the language of establishing "confidence." Jay Forrester and Peter Senge discussed tests for
building confidence. They write pithily that:

> It is pointless to try to establish that a particular model is useful
> without specifying *for what purpose* it is to be used. (Forrester and
> Senge, 1996, p. 8)[3]

The authors were also explicit about the many *types* of use to which
models can be put. For example, they refer to pattern prediction—i.e.,
whether a model generates *qualitatively* correct patterns of future
behavior relating to periods, phases, or changes (Forrester and Senge,
1996, p. 23) or whether the model reports on the potential for events
to occur, such as rapid depletion of a resource or rapid rise in prices of
some commodity (p. 24). Especially relevant is anticipating surprise
behaviors (p. 26). When this occurs with system models, it sometimes
identifies risks to the real system that had previously not been recognized. Forrester and Senge had in mind what we have called exploratory
analysis and coarse prediction in our report. A model may be valuable
for those even if it does not make accurate and precise predictions.

A more recent paper from the system dynamics literature muses
about how SD models are not always accepted and suggests distinguishing them on a simple scale that amounts to assigning them a qualitative

---

[3]   Such early papers demonstrate how long the issues have been recognized. A better modern
source is John Sterman's comprehensive textbook (Sterman, 2000), including its candid discussion of how models can be "protective" (covering up) or "reflective" (p. 858).

type of validity—i.e., describing "levels of evidence" supporting the model (Homer, 2014).

Model validity has also been discussed in the context of dealing with "soft" models and with models used for what RAND has variously called exploratory modeling and exploratory analysis (Davis and Finch, 1993; Davis, 1994; Bigelow and Davis, 2003; Bankes, 1993). Such analysis is crucial for planning strategies intended to be flexible, adaptive, and robust (FARness) (Davis, 2014) or, in alternative language, seeking to aid robust decisionmaking (RDM) (Lempert et al., 2006). In the latter usage, "robust" is shorthand covering the several attributes.

A 2011 workshop at Sandia National Laboratories had much to say about validation, particularly about the need to recognize that, at least in social-behavioral modeling, one should not look to models specifically for prediction, forecasting, or other synonyms (McNamara et al., 2011). A background paper by Jessica Turnley reviewed the issue and had some delightful language at the end relating exploratory analysis to the reading of great literature:

> Our argument is based on the claim that computational social models are inherently unable to be used for predictive purposes in the same way that models of physical and many biological phenomena can. Ethical issues, the complex nature of the socio-cultural domain, the nature of the data, and the inherent time scales of the phenomena under consideration severely constrain the types, breadth and depth of experiments we can conduct to ascertain predictive capability. At best, computational social models can rely upon the (proxy) validity of the narrative theory upon which they are based.
>
> That said, there are other means of ascertaining goodness. All computational models are built with a use in mind. If we broaden our thinking and consider ways other than prediction to use computational social models, we will begin to realize alternative means of assessing their goodness.
>
> The question of degree of isomorphism to the "real world" (or target domain) may become moot. Just as we continue to read Goethe although we never expect to actually meet Faust, so might we build and use computational social models although

**Figure C.1**
**Spider Charts for Multifaceted Characterization of Model Validity**

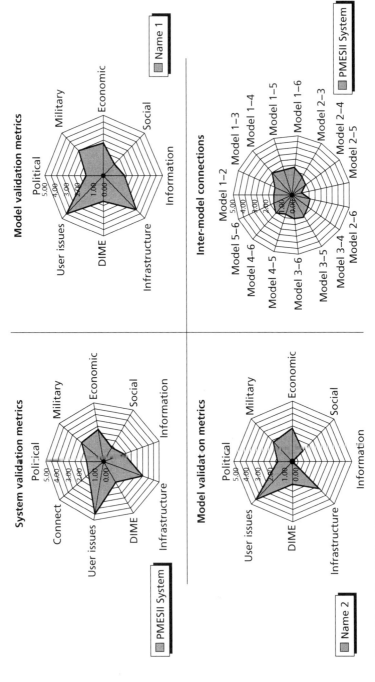

SOURCE: Hartley, 2010, p. 330.

we never expect to actually live in the future any one of them "predicts." Although not accurate, computational social models can still be useful—and, even better, true. (Turnley, 2011, pp. 241–254)

In recent times, Dean Hartley and Stuart Starr studied how to conduct VV&A, and then describe results for DoD models addressing political, military, economic, social, infrastructure, and information issues (PMESII). They introduced a categorical scale (from uncodified to fully validated) and then applied it separately to the PMESII components of the models in question. Figure C.1 is an example (Hartley, 2010, p. 330). The message from the examples is that, for the models in question, most rated poorly on substantive grounds (perhaps 1 on a 1–5 scale), but some did well in "practical" ways, such as user-friendliness and shareability. The study did not intend to break new ground in understanding what validity means, but rather to show how simple and subjective measurements, along with important distinctions, could lead to multifaceted model assessments understandable at a glance.

# Participants in Workshops

A workshop on science and modeling of social and behavioral issues was held in RAND's Santa Monica, California, office on April 3–4, 2017, combining what had previously been planned as two separate workshops. Table D.1 lists the participants. Their backgrounds or current research involve at least the following areas: anthropology, chemical physics, complexity sciences, computer science physics, communication, control and dynamical systems, economics, geography, industrial and systems engineering law, mathematics, history, behavioral biology, electrical engineering, law, political science, psychology, sociology, social systems science, and technology. Most cross disciplines.

**Table D.1**
**Participants in Workshop on Social-Behavioral Modeling and Simulation**

| Name | Affiliation |
| --- | --- |
| Karyn Apfeldorf | Areté Associates |
| Robert Axtell | George Mason University |
| Matthew Brashears | University of South Carolina |
| Kathleen Carley | Carnegie Mellon University |
| Steven Corman | Arizona State University |
| Paul Davis | RAND and Pardee RAND Graduate School |
| Richard Davis | Artis Research & Risk Modeling |
| Simon DeDeo | Carnegie Mellon and the Sante Fe Institute |
| Charles Ehlschlaeger | U.S. Army Corps of Engineers |
| Joshua Epstein | Johns Hopkins University |
| Dana Eyre | SoSACorp |

**Table D.1—Continued**

| Name | Affiliation |
| --- | --- |
| Jessica Flack | Sante Fe Institute |
| Michael Gabbay | University of Washington |
| Lise Getoor | University of California, Santa Cruz |
| Timothy Gulden | RAND |
| Ali Jadbabaie | Massachusetts Institute of Technology |
| Brian Jenkins | RAND |
| Melvin Konner | Emory University |
| Bart Kosko | University of Southern California |
| David Krakauer | Sante Fe Institute |
| Kiran Lakkaraju | Sandia National Laboratories |
| Alexander Levis | George Mason University |
| Corey Lofdahl | SoSACorp |
| Christian Madsbjerg | ReD Associates |
| Lynn Miller | University of Southern California |
| Kent Myers | Office of the Director or National Intelligence |
| Benjamin Nyblade | University of California, Los Angeles |
| Angela O'Mahony | RAND and Pardee RAND Graduate School |
| Osonde Osoba | RAND |
| Edward Palazzolo | Army Research Office |
| Jonathan Pfautz | Defense Advanced Research Agency |
| Hazhir Rahmandad | Massachusetts Institute of Technology |
| William Rand | North Carolina State University |
| Stephen Read | University of Southern California |
| William Rouse | Stevens Institute of Technology |
| Philip Schrodt | Parus Analytics |
| Katharine Sieck | RAND |
| Amy Sliva | Charles River Associates |
| Samarth Swarup | Virginia Tech |
| Leigh Tesfatsion | Iowa State University |
| Andreas Tolk | MITRE |
| Rand Waltzman | RAND |
| Levent Yilmaz | Auburn University |
| Michael Zyda | University of Southern California |

# Abbreviations

We have tried to minimize dependence on acronyms in this report, but the table below shows the ones that appear.

| Acronym | Meaning |
|---|---|
| ABM | agent-based modeling |
| CAS | complex adaptive systems |
| DARPA | Defense Advanced Research Projects Agency |
| DoD | Department of Defense |
| EA and EM | exploratory analysis and exploratory modeling (roughly synonymous) |
| FARness | flexibility, adaptiveness, and robustness |
| HSCB | Human, Social and Culture Behavior Modeling |
| IoE | Internet of Everything |
| M&S | modeling and simulation |
| MRM and MRMPM | multiresolution modeling; multiresolution, multiperspective modeling |
| MS&A | modeling, simulation, and analysis |
| NRC | National Research Council |
| RDM | robust decisionmaking |
| SB | social-behavioral |
| SBML | social-behavioral modeling laboratory |
| SD | system dynamics |
| V&V and VV&A | verification, validation, and accreditation |

# References

Abdollahian, Mark, Michael Barnick, Brian Efird, and Jacek Kugler (2006), *Senturion: A Predictive Political Simulation Model,* Washington, D.C.: National Defense University.

Adams, Marvin L., and David M. Hidden (2012), *Assessing the Reliability of Complex Models: Mathematical and Statistical Foundations of Verification, Validation, and Uncertainty Quantification*, Washington, D.C.: National Academies Press.

Agar, Michael (2013), *The Lively Science: Remodeling Human Social Research*, Minneapolis, Minn.: Mill City Press.

Albro, Robert (2011), "Mining Sentiments: Computational Modeling and the Interpretive Problem of Culture," in *Challenges in Computational Social Modeling and Simulation for National Security Decision-Making*, edited by Laura A. McNamara, Timothy G. Trucano, and Charles Gieseler, Albuquerque, N.M.: Sandia National Laboratories, 83–108.

Angrist, Joshua D., and Jorn-Steffen Pischke (2009), *Mostly Harmless Econometrics: An Empiricist's Companion*, Princeton, N.J.: Princeton University Press.

Angwin, Julia, and Jeff Larson (2017), "Bias in Criminal Risk Scores Is Mathematically Inevitable, Researchers Say." https://www.propublica.org/article/bias-in-criminal-risk-scores-is-mathematically -inevitable-researchers-say (accessed November 25, 2017).

Atran, Scott (2010), *Talking to the Enemy: Faith, Brotherhood, and the Unmaking of Terrorists*, New York: Harper Collins Publishers.

Atran, Scott, and Robert Axelrod (2008), "In Theory: Reframing Sacred Values," *Negotiation Journal*, July, 221–245.

Axelrod, Robert (1997), *The Complexity of Cooperation: Agent-Based Models of Competition and Collaboration*, Princeton, N.J.: Princeton University Press.

Balebako, Rebecca, Angela O'Mahony, Paul K. Davis, and Osonde A. Osoba (2017), *Lessons from a Workshop on Ethical and Privacy Issues in Social-Behavioral Research,* PR-2867, Santa Monica, Calif.: RAND Corporation.

Bankes, Steven C. (1993), "Exploratory Modeling for Policy Analysis," *Operations Research*, 41 (3), 435–449.

Bar-Yam, Yaneer (1997), *Dynamics of Complex Systems*, Reading, Mass.: Perseus Books.

Berrebi, Claude (2009), "The Economics of Terrorism and Counterterrorism: What Matters and Is Rational-Choice Theory Helpful?," in *Social Science for Counterterrorism: Putting the Pieces Together*, edited by Paul K. Davis and Kim Cragin, Santa Monica, Calif.: RAND Corporation, 151–208.

Berrebi, Claude, and Darius Lakdawalla (2007), "How Does Terrorism Risk Vary Across Space and Time? An Analysis Based on the Israeli Experience," *Defence and Peace Economics*, 18 (2), 113–131.

Bigelow, James H., and Paul K. Davis (2003), *Implications for Model Validation of Multiresolution, Multiperspective Modeling (MRMPM), and Exploratory Analysis*, Santa Monica, Calif.: RAND Corporation, MR-1570-AF.

Blaha, Michael, and James Rumbaugh (2005), *Object-Oriented Modeling and Design with UML*, 2nd ed., Upper Saddle River, N.J.: Pearson Prentice Hall.

Boehm, Barry, and Wilfred J. Hansen (2000), *Serial Development, Experience, Principles, and Refinements,* CMU/SEI-2000-SR-008, Pittsburgh, Penn.: Carnegie Mellon Software Engineering Institute.

Bookstaber, Richard (2017), *The End of Theory: Financial Crises, the Failure of Economics, and the Sweep of Human Interactions*, Princeton, N.J.: Princeton University Press.

Box, George E. P. (2000), *Statistics for Discovery*, Report No. 179, Madison, Wisc.: Center for Quality and Productivity, University of Wisconsin.

Brashears, Matthew E., and David L. Sallach (2014), "Modeling Cognitions, Networks, Strategic Games, and Ecologies," in *Sociocultural Behavior Sensemaking: State of the Art in Understanding the Operational Environment,* edited by Jill D. Egeth, Gary L. Klein, and Dylan Schmorrow, McLean, Virg.: MITRE, 29–50.

Breiger, Ron, Kathleen M. Carley, and Phillippa Pattison, eds. (2003), *Dynamic Social Network Modeling and Analysis*, Washington, D.C.: National Academies Press.

Bueno de Mesquita, Bruce (1983), *The War Trap*, New Haven, Conn.: Yale University Press.

———— (2010), *The Predictioneer's Game: Using the Logic of Brazen Self-Interest to See and Shape the Future*, New York: Random House Trade Paperbacks.

Carley, Kathleen M. (2006), "Appendix B: Social Behavioral Modeling," in *Defense Modeling, Simulation, and Analysis: Meeting the Challenge*, Washington, D.C.: National Academies Press, 64–73.

———— (2012), "Deterrence Modeling Using Dynamic Network Analysis," briefing, Pittsburgh: Carnegie Mellon University, Center for Computational Analysis of Social and Organizational Systems.

Carlson, James, Arthur Jaffe, and Andrew Wiles, eds. (2006), *The Millennium Prize Problems*, Providence, R.I.: American Mathematical Society.

Cartwright, Nancy (1983), *How the Laws of Physics Lie*, Oxford: Oxford University Press.

———— (1999), *The Dappled World: A Study of the Boundaries of Science*, Cambridge: Cambridge University Press.

———— (2004), "Causation: One Word, Many Things," *Philosophy of Science*, 71 (5).

Čavojová, Vladimira (2018), "When Beliefs and Logic Contradict: Issues of Values, Religion, and Culture," in *Advances in Culturally-Aware Intelligent Systems and in Cross-Cultural Psychological Studies*, edited by Colette Faucher, Cham, Switzerland: Springer International, 367–390.

Churchman, Charles W. (1967), "Wicked Problems," *Management Science*, 14 (4), B-141.

Confessore, Nicholas, and Danny Hakim (2017), "Data Firm Says 'Secret Sauce' Aided Trump; Many Scoff," *New York Times*, March 6. https://www.nytimes.com/2017/03/06/us/politics/cambridge-analytica.html?mcubz = 3&_r = 0

Corman, Steven R. N. (2012), "Understanding Sociocultural Systems Through a Narrative Lens," in *A Sociocultural Systems Primer for the Military Thinker: Multidisciplinary Perspectives and Approaches*, edited by L. Brooks et al., Leavenworth, Kans.: U.S. Army Research Institute, 71–86.

Davis, Paul K. (1989), *Some Lessons Learned from Building Red Agents in the RAND Strategy Assessment System,* Santa Monica, Calif.: RAND Corporation, N-3003-OSD.

————, ed. (1994), *New Challenges in Defense Planning: Rethinking How Much Is Enough*, Santa Monica, Calif.: RAND Corporation.

———— (2003), "Exploratory Analysis and Implications for Modeling," in *New Challenges, New Tools*, edited by Stuart Johnson, Martin Libicki, and Gregory Treverton, Santa Monica, Calif.: RAND Corporation, 255–283.

————, ed. (2011), *Dilemmas of Intervention: Social Science for Stabilization and Reconstruction*, Santa Monica, Calif.: RAND Corporation.

———— (2012), *Some Lessons from RAND's Work on Planning Under Uncertainty for National Security*, Santa Monica, Calif.: RAND Corporation, TR-1429-OSD.

———— (2014), *Analysis to Inform Defense Planning Despite Austerity*, Santa Monica, Calif.: RAND Corporation.

———— (2016), *Capabilities for Joint Analysis in the Department of Defense: Rethinking Support for Strategic Analysis*, Santa Monica, Calif.: RAND Corporation.

———— (2017), "Illustrating a Model-Game-Model Paradigm for Using Human Wargames in Analysis," Santa Monica, Calif.: RAND Corporation, WP-1179.

Davis, Paul K., and Robert H. Anderson (2003), *Improving the Composability of Department of Defense Models and Simulations*, Santa Monica, Calif.: RAND Corporation.

Davis, Paul K., Steven C. Bankes, and Michael Egner (2007), *Enhancing Strategic Planning with Massive Scenario Generation: Theory and Experiments,* Santa Monica, Calif.: RAND Corporation, TR-392-OSD.

Davis, Paul K., and James H. Bigelow (1998), *Experiments in Multiresolution Modeling (MRM)*, Santa Monica, Calif.: RAND Corporation, MR-1004-DARPA.

———— (2003), *Motivated Metamodels: Synthesis of Cause-Effect Reasoning and Statistical Metamodeling*, Santa Monica, Calif.: RAND Corporation.

Davis, Paul K., and Kim Cragin, eds. (2009), *Social Science for Counterterrorism: Putting the Pieces Together*, Santa Monica, Calif.: RAND Corporation.

Davis, Paul K., and Lou Finch (1993), *Defense Planning in the Post–Cold War Era: Giving Meaning to Flexibility, Adaptiveness, and Robustness of Capability*, Santa Monica, Calif.: RAND Corporation.

Davis, Paul K., and Richard Hillestad (1993), "Families of Models That Cross Levels of Resolution: Issues for Design, Calibration, and Management," in *Proceedings of the 1993 Winter Simulation Conference*, edited by G. W. Evans et al., Society for Computer Simulation, 1003–1012.

Davis, Paul K., Eric Larson, Zachary Haldeman, Mustafa Oquz, and Yasholdhara Rana (2012), *Understanding and Influencing Public Support for Insurgency and Terrorism*, Santa Monica, Calif.: RAND Corporation.

Davis, Paul K., and Angela O'Mahony (2013), *A Computational Model of Public Support for Insurgency and Terrorism: A Prototype for More General Social-Science Modeling*, Santa Monica, Calif.: RAND Corporation, TR-1220.

———— (2017), "Representing Qualitative Social Science in Computational Models to Aid Reasoning Under Uncertainty: National Security Examples," *Journal of Defense Modeling and Simulation*, 14 (1), 1–22.

Davis, Paul K., Walter L. Perry, John S. Hollywood, and David Manheim (2016), *Uncertainty-Sensitive Heterogeneous Information Fusion: Assessing Threat with Soft, Uncertain, and Conflicting Evidence*, Santa Monica, Calif.: RAND Corporation.

Davis, Paul K., and James A. Winnefeld (1983), *The RAND Corp. Strategy Assessment Center*, Santa Monica, Calif.: RAND Corporation, R-3535-NA.

Davis, Richard (2016), *Hamas, Popular Support, and War in the Middle East*, London and New York: Routledge.

DeDeo, Simon, David C. Krakauer, and Jessica C. Flack (2010), "Inductive Game Theory and the Dynamics of Armed Conflict," *PLoS Computational Biology*, 6 (5), 1–16.

Defense Modeling and Simulation Coordination Office (DM&SCO) (2016), "M&S Glossary." https://www.msco.mil/MSReferences/Glossary/MSGlossary.aspx (accessed December 1, 2017).

Della Vigna, Stefano, and Ulrike Malmender (2006), "Paying Not to Go to the Gym," *American Economic Review*, 96 (3), 694–719.

Department of Defense (2009), *DoD Modeling and Simulation (M&S) Verification, Validation, and Accreditation (VV&A)*, Number 5000.61.

Diamond, Jared (1987), "Soft Sciences Are Often Harder Than Hard Sciences," *Discover*, 8, 34–39.

Dirac, Paul Adrien Maurice (1939), "The Relation Between Mathematics and Physics," *Proceedings of the Royal Society of Edinburgh*, 59, Part II, 122–129.

Dobson, Geoffrey B., and Kathleen M. Carley (2017), "Cyber-Fit: An Agent-Based Modelling Approach to Simulating Cyber Warfare," in *10th International Conference on Social Computing, Behavioral-Cultural Modeling and Prediction and Behavior Representation (SBP-BriMS) in Modeling and Simulation*, edited by D. Lee, Y. R. Lin, N. Osgood, and R. Thomson, 139–148.

Dörner, Dietrich (1997), *The Logic of Failure: Recognizing and Avoiding Errors in Complex Situations*, Cambridge, Mass.: Perseus Books.

Dorratoltaj, Nargesalsadat, Achla Marathe, Bryan L. Lewis, Samarth Swarup, Stephen G. Eubank, and Kaja M. Abbas (2017), "Epidemiological and Economic Impact of Pandemic Influenza in Chicago: Priorities for Vaccine intervention," *PLoS Computational Biology*, 13 (6): e1005521. https://doi.org/10.1371/journal.pcbi.1005521

Dreyer, Paul, Edward Balkovich, and David Manheim (2016), "Modeling the Secuity and Resilience of a Coupled Economic System Using High-Performance Computing with MAQUETTES," PR-2703-RC.

Egeth, Jill D., Gary L. Klein, and Dylan Schmorrow, eds. (2014), *Sociocultural Behavior Sensemaking: State of the Art in Understanding the Operational Environment*, McLean, Va.: MITRE.

Ehlschlaeger, Charles R. (2002), "Representing Multiple Spatial Statistics in Generalized Elevation Uncertainty Models: Moving Beyond the Variogram," *International Journal of Geographical Information Science*, 16 (3), 259–285.

Ehlschlaeger, Charles R., Ashton M. Shortridge, and Michael F. Goodchild (1997), "Visualizing Spatial Data Uncertainty Using Animation," *Computers and Geosciences*, 23(4), 387–395.

Elsaesser, Chris, et al. (2014), "Computational Sociocultural Models Used for Forecasting," in *Sociocultural Behavior Sensemaking: State of the Art in Understanding the Operational Environment*, edited by Jill D. Egeth, Gary L. Klein, and Dylan Schmorrow, McLean, Virg.: MITRE, 269–314.

Elson, Sara Beth, Alison Dingwall, and Mansoor Moaddel (2014), "Sociocultural Approaches to Understand Human Interaction: A Discussion of New Theoretical Frameworks, Issues, and Modern Communication Technology," in *Sociocultural Behavior Sensemaking: State of the Art in Understanding the Operational Environment*, edited by Jill D. Egeth, Gary L. Klein, and Dylan Schnorrow, McLean, Virg.: MITRE, 9–28.

Epstein, Joshua M. (1999), "Agent-Based Computational Models and Generative Social Science," *Complexity*, 4 (5), 41–60.

———— (2014), *Agent_Zero: Toward Neurcognitive Foundations for Generative Social Science*, Princeton, N.J.: Princeton University Press.

Epstein, Joshua M., and Robert L. Axtell (1996), *Growing Artificial Societies: Social Science from the Bottom Up*, Cambridge, Mass.: MIT Press.

Eyre, Dana P., and James R. Littleton (2012), "Shaping the Zeitgeist: Influencing Social Processes as the Center of Gravity for Strategic Communications in the Twenty-First Century," *Public Relations Review*, 38, 179–187.

Farnadi, Bolnoosh, Stephen H. Bach, Marie-Francine Moens, Lise Getoor, and Martine de Cock (2017), "Soft Quantification in Statistical Relational Learning," *Machine Learning Journal*, 1–21.

Faucher, Colette, ed. (2018), *Advances in Culturally-Aware Intelligent Systems and in Cross-Cultural Psychological Studies*, Paris: Springer International.

Feyerabend, Paul (1975), *Against Method*, with Introduction by Ian Hacking, New York and London: Verso.

Financial Crisis Inquiry Commission (2011), *Financial Crisis Inquiry Report*, Washington, D.C.: GPO.

Fischbach, Jordan R. (2010), "Managing New Orleans Flood Risk in an Uncertain Future Using Non-Structural Risk Mitigation," dissertation, Santa Monica, Calif.: Pardee RAND Graduate School.

Fishwick, Paul A. (2004), "Toward an Integrative Multimodeling Interface: A Human-Computer Interface Approach to Interrelating Model Structures," *SCS Trans Model Simul*, 80 (9), 421–432.

Fishwick, Paul A., and Bernard P. Zeigler (1992), "A Multimodel Methodology for Qualitative Model Engineering," *ACM Transactions on Modeling and Computer Simulations*, 2 (1), 52–81.

Flack, Jessica C. (2012), "Multiple Time-Scales and the Developmental Dynamics of Social Systems," *Philosophical Transactions of the Royal Society B*, 367 (1597), 1802–1810.

Flack, Jessica C., and Frans B. M. de Waal (2000), " 'Any Animal Whatever': Darwinian Building Blocks of Morality in Monkeys and Apes," *Journal of Consciousness Studies*, 7 (1–2), 1–29.

Flack, Jessica C., Frans B. M. de Waal, and David C. Krakauer (2005), "Social Structure, Robustness, and Policing Cost in a Cognitively Sophisticated Species," *The American Naturalist*, 165 (5).

Flyvbjerg, Bent (2001), *Making Social Science Matter: Why Social Inquiry Fails and How It Can Succeed Again*, Cambridge, UK: Cambridge University Press.

———— (2004), "A Perestroikan Straw Man Answers Back: David Laitin and Phronetic Political Science," *Politics & Society*, 32 (3), 389–416.

Flyvbjerg, Bent, and Todd Landman, eds. (2012), *Real Social Science: Applied Phronesis*, Cambridge, U.K.: Cambridge University Press.

Forrester, Jay W. (1963), *Industrial Dynamics*, Cambridge, Mass.: MIT Press.

Forrester, Jay W., and Peter M. Senge (1996), "Tests for Building Confidence in System Dynamic Models," in *Modelling for Management Simulation in Support of Systems Thinking, Vol. 2*, edited by George P. Richardson, Aldershot, England: Dartmouth Publishing, 414–434.

Forrester, Jay Wright (1969), *Urban Dynamics*, Cambridge, Mass.: Wright Allen Press.

Fricker, Ronald D., Samuel E. Buttrey, and William Evans (2014), "Visualization for Sociocultural Signature Detection," in *Sociocultural Behavior Sensemaking: State of the Art in Understanding the Operational Environment*, edited by Jill D. Egeth, Gary L. Klein, and Dylan Schmorrow, McLean, Virg.: MITRE, 173–216.

Friedman, Jerome H., and Nicholas I. Fisher (1999), "Bump Hunting in High-Dimensional Data," *Statistics and Computing*, 9 (2), 123–143.

Gabbay, Michael (2014), "Data Processing for Applications of Dynamics-Based Models to Forecasting," in *Sociocultural Behavior Sensemaking: State of the Art in Understanding the Operational Environment*, edited by Jill D. Egeth, Gary L. Klein, and Dylan Schmorrow, McLean, Virg.: MITRE, 245–269.

George, Alexander L., and Andrew Bennett (2005), *Case Studies and Theory Development in the Social Sciences*, Cambridge, Mass.: MIT Press.

Gilbert, Daniel T., Gary King, Stephen Pettigrew, and Timothy D. Wilson (2016), "Comment on 'Estimating the Reproducibility of Psychological Science,' " *Science*, 351 (6277), 1037.

Grimm, Volker, Uta Berger, Donald L. DeAngelis, J. Gary Polhill, Jarl Giske, and Steven F. Railsback (2010), "The ODD Protocol: A Review and First Update," *Ecological Modelling*, 221, 2760–2768.

Groves, David G., and Robert J. Lempert (2007), "A New Analytic Method for Finding Policy-Relevant Scenarios," *Global Environmental Change*, 17(1), 78–85.

Groves, David G., Christopher Sharon, and Debra Knopman (2013), *Planning Tool to Support Louisiana's Decisionmaking on Coastal Protection and Restoration: Technical Description*, Santa Monica, Calif.: RAND Corporation.

Haack, Susan (2011), *Defending Science—Within Reason: Between Scientism and Cynicism*, Amherst, N. Y.: Prometheus Books.

Haasnoot, Marjolijn, Jan H. Kwakkel, Warren E. Walker, and Judith Ter Maat (2013), "Dynamic Adaptive Policy Pathways: a Method for Crafting Robust Decisions for a Deeply Uncertain World," *Global Environmental Change,* 23 (2), 435–498.

Hadzikadic, Mirsad, Sean O'Brien, and Khouja Moufaz, eds. (2013), *Managing Complexity: Practical Considerations in the Development and Application of ABMs to Contemporary Policy Challenges*, Springer International.

Haidt, Jonathan (2013), *The Righteous Mind: Why Good People Are Divided by Politics and Religion*, New York: Vintage.

Halpern, Joseph Y. (2016), *Actual Causality*, Cambridge, Mass.: MIT Press.

Halverson, Jeffry R., H. Lloyd Goodall, and Steven C. Corman (2011), *Master Narratives of Islamist Extremism*, New York: Palgrave-MacMillan.

Hardt, Moritz, Eric Price, and Nathan Srebo (2017), "Equality of Opportunity in Supervised Learning," *ARXIV*, eprint arXiv:1610.02413.

Hart, Vi, and Nicky Case (undated), "Parable of the Polygons." http://ncase.me/polygons/ (accessed August 30, 2017).

Hartley, Dean (2010), "Comparing Validation Results for Two DIME/PMESII Models: Understanding Coverage Profiles," *Proceedings of the 2010 Winter Simulation Conference*, edited by B. Johansson et al., IEEE, 428–440.

Herman, Mark L., and Mark D. Frost (2009), *Wargaming for Leaders: Strategic Decision Making from the Battlefield to the Boardroom*, McLean, Virg.: Booz Allen Hamilton.

Hethcote, Herbert W. (2000), "The Mathematics of Infectious Diseases," *SIAM Review*, 42 (4), 599–653.

Holland, John H. (1998), *Emergence: From Chaos to Order*, Cambridge, Mass.: Perseus Books.

Holland, John H., and Heather Mimnaugh (1996), *Hidden Order: How Adaptation Builds Complexity*, New York: Perseus Publishing.

Homer, Jack (2014), "Levels of Evidence in System Dynamics Modeling," *System Dynamics Review*, 30 (1–2), 75–80.

Homer, Jack B., and Gary B. Hirsch (2006), "System Dynamics Modeling for Public Health: Background and Opportunities," *American Journal of Public Health*, 96 (3), 452–458.

Hruschka, Daniel (2010), *Friendship: Development, Ecology, and Evolution*, Berkeley and Los Angeles: University of California Press.

Irvine, John M. (2014), "Transforming Data into Information: Enabling Detection and Discovery for Sociocultural Analysis," in *Sociocultural Behavior Sensemaking: State of the Art in Understanding the Operational Environment*, edited by Jill D. Egeth, Gary L. Klein, and Dylan Schmorrow, McLean, Virg.: MITRE, 111–146.

Issenberg, Sasha (2012), *The Victory Lab: The Secret Science of Winning Campaigns*, New York: Crown.

Jenkins, Brian Michael (2017), *The Origin of America's Jihadists*, Santa Monica, Calif.: RAND Corporation, PE-251-RC.

Jervis, Robert (1976), *Perception and Misperception in International Politics*, Princeton, N.J.: Princeton University Press.

Jima, Lee, and Kira Lakkaraju (2014), "Predicting Social Ties in Massively Multiplayer Online Games," in *International Conference on Social Computing, Behavioral-Cultural Modeling, and Prediction (SBP14)*, edited by William Kennedy, Nitin Agerwal, and Shanchieh Jay Yang Springer, 95–102.

Kalyvas, Stathis N. (2008), "Promises and Pitfalls of an Emerging Research Program: The Microdynamics of Civil War," in *Order, Conflict, and Violence*, edited by Stathis N. Kalyvas, Ian Shapiro, and Tarek Masoud, New York: Cambridge University Press, 397–421.

Kaplan, Abraham (1964), *The Conduct of Inquiry: Methodology for Behavioral Science*, San Francisco, Calif.: Chandler Publishing Company.

Knorr-Cetina, Karin (1999), *Epistemic Cultures: How the Sciences Make Knowledge*, Cambridge, Mass.: Harvard University Press.

Konner, Melvin (2003), *The Tangled Wing: Biological Constraints on the Human Spirit,* New York: Henry Holt and Company.

——— (2015), "The Weather of Violence: Metaphors and Models, Predictions and Surprises," *Counter-Terrorism Exchange (CTX)*, 5 (3), 53–64.

Koonin, Steven E. (2014), "Climate Science Is Not Settled," *Wall Street Journal*, The Saturday Essay, https://www.wsj.com/articles/climate-science-is-not-settled-1411143565

Kött, Alexander, and Gary Citrenbaum, eds. (2010), *Estimating Impact: A Handbook of Computational Methods and Models for Anticipating Economic, Social, Political, and Security Effects in International Interventions*, New York: Springer.

Kuhn, Thomas (1970), *The Structure of Scientific Revolutions*, Cambridge, Mass.: MIT Press.

Kuznar, Lawrence A. (2008), *Reclaiming a Scientific Anthropology*, 2nd ed., New York: AltaMira Press.

Laitin, David D. (2003), "The Perestroikan Challenge to Social Science," *Politics & Society*, 31 (1), 163–184.

Lempert, Robert J., David G. Groves, Steven W. Popper, and Steven C. Bankes (2006), "A General Analytic Method for Generating Robust Strategies and Narrative Scenarios," *Management Science*, 4 (April), 514–528.

Lempert, Robert J., Steven W. Popper, and Steven C. Bankes (2003), *Shaping the Next One Hundred Years: New Methods for Quantitative Long-Term Policy Analysis*, Santa Monica, Calif.: RAND Corporation.

Lende, Daniel H. (2012), "Poverty Poisons the Brain," *Annals of Anthropological Practice*, 36 (1), 183–201.

Leveror, Robert H. (2016), "Crowds as Complex Adaptive Systems: Strategic Implications for Law Enforcement," dissertation, Monterey, Calif.: U.S. Naval Postgraduate School.

Levis, Alexander H. (2016), "Multi-Formalism Modeling of Human Organization," in *Seminal Contributions to Modeling and Simulation*, edited by K. Al-Begain and A. Bargiela, Basel, Switzerland: Springer International, 23–46.

Levis, Alexander H., Lee W. Wagenhals, and Abbas K. Zaidi (2010), "Multi-Modeling of Adversary Behaviors," in *IEEE International Conference on Intelligence and Security Informatics (ISI), Vancouver*, IEEE, 185–189.

Lewis, Michael (2010), *The Big Short: Inside the Doomsday Machine*, New York: W. W. Norton.

Lofdahl, Corey (2001), *Environmental Impacts of Globalization and Trade*, Cambridge, Mass.: MIT Press.

——— (2010), "Governance and Society," in *Estimating Impact*, edited by Alexander Kott and Gary Citrenbaum, New York: Springer, 179–204.

Lustick, Ian S. (2014), "Making Sense of Social Radar: V-Saft as an Intelligent Machine," in *Sociocultural Behavior Sensemaking: State of the Art in Understanding the Operational Environment*, edited by Jill D. Egeth, Gary L. Klein, and Dylan Schmorrow, McLean, Virg.: MITRE, 317–338.

Madsbjerg, Christian (2017), *Sensemaking: The Power of the Humanities in the Age of the Algorithm*, New York: Hachette Books.

Matsumura, John, Randal Steeb, John Gordon, Tom Herbert, Russell Glenn, and Paul Steinberg. (2001), *Lightning over Water: Sharpening America's Capabilities for Rapid-Reaction Missions*, Santa Monica, Calif.: RAND Corporation.

McNamara, Laura A., Timothy G. Trucano, and Charles Gieseler, eds. (2011), *Challenges in Computational Social Modeling and Simulation for National Security Decision-Making*, OSRD 2011 002, Albuquerque, N.M.: Sandia National Laboratories.

Mehlhase, Alexandra (2014), "A Python Framework to Create and Simulate Models with Variable Structure in Common Simulation Environments," *Mathematical and Computer Modeling of Dynamical Systems*, November.

Mingers, John, and Anthony Gill, eds. (1997), *Multimethodology: The Theory and Practice of Combining Management Science Methodologies*, Chichester, England: John Wiley & Sons.

Nardi, Bonnie E., ed. (1996), *Context and Consciousness: Activity Theory and Human-Computer Interaction*, Cambridge, Mass.: MIT Press.

National Research Council (1997), *Modeling and Simulation, Vol. 9 of Technology for the United States Navy and Marine Corps: 2000–2035*, Washington, D.C.: Naval Studies Board, National Academy Press.

——— (2006), *Defense Modeling, Simulation, and Analysis: Meeting the Challenge*, Washington, D.C.: National Academies Press.

——— (2010), *The Rise of Games and High-Performance Computing for Modeling and Simulation*, Washington, D.C.: National Academies Press.

——— (2014), *U.S. Air Force Strategic Deterrence Analytic Capabilities: An Assessment of Methods, Tools, and Approaches for the 21st Century Security Environment*, Washington, D.C.: National Academies Press.

National Research Council, and Robert Pool, rapporteur (2011), *Sociocultural Data to Accomplish Department of Defense Missions: Toward a Unified Social Framework: Workshop Summary*, Washington, D.C.: National Academies Press.

Nickerson, David W., and Todd Rogers (2014), "Political Campaigns and Big Data," *Journal of Economic Perspectives*, 28 (2), 51–73.

Nicolis, Gregoire, and Ilya Prigogine (1977), *Self-Organization in Nonequilibrium Systems: From Dissipative Structures to Order Through Fluctuations*, New York: John Wiley & Sons.

Noricks, Darcy M. E. (2009), "The Root Causes of Terrorism," in *Social Science for Counterterrorism; Putting the Pieces Together*, edited by Paul K. Davis and Kim Cragin, Santa Monica, Calif.: RAND Corporation, 11–70.

North, Michael J., and Charles M. Macal (2007), *Managing Business Complexity: Discovering Strategic Solutions with Agent-Based Modeling and Simulation*, New York: Oxford University Press.

Nyblade, Benjamin, Angela O'Mahony, and Katharinee Sieck (2017), *State of Social and Behavioral Science Theories*, Santa Monica, Calif.: RAND Corporation, PR-3002-DARPA.

Olabisi, Laura Schmitt, Ryan Qi Wang, and Arika Ligmann-Zielinska (2015), "Why Don't More Farmers Go Organic? Using a Stakeholder-Informed Exploratory Agent-Based Model to Represent the Dynamics of Farming Practices in the Philippines," *Land*, 4 (4): 979–1002.

Open Science Collaboration (2015), "Estimating the Reproducibility of Psychological Science," *Science*, 349 (6251).

Osoba, Osonde, and Paul K. Davis (forthcoming), *An Artificial Intelligence/ Machine Learning Perspective on Social Simulation: New Data and New Challenges*, Santa Monica, Calif.: RAND Corporation, WR-1213.

Osoba, Osonde, and Bart Kosko (2017), "Fuzzy Knowledge Fusion for Causal Modeling," *Journal of Defense Modeling and Simulation*, 14 (1), 17–32.

Pace, Dale K. (2004), "Modeling and Simulation Verification and Validation Challenges," *Johns Hopkins Applied Physics Laboratory Technical Digest*, 25 (2).

Page, Scott E. (2010), *Diversity and Complexity (Primers in Complex Systems)*, Princeton, N.J.: Princeton University Press.

Parikh, Nidhi, Madhav Marathe, and Samarth Swarup (2016), "Summarizing Simulation Results Using Causally Relevant States," in *International Conference on Autonomous Agents and Multiagent Systems (AAMAS 2016): Autonomous Agents and Multiagent Systems*, edited by N. Osman and C. Sierra, Springer, 88–103.

Pearl, Judea (2009a), "Causal Inference in Statistics: An Overview," *Statistics Surveys*, R-350.

——— (2009b), *Causality: Models, Reasoning, and Inference*, Cambridge, Mass.: Cambridge University Press.

Peirce, Charles S. (1877), "The Fixation of Belief," *Popular Science Monthly*, 12, 1–15.

Peirce, Charles S., and Justus Buchler, eds. (1940), *Philosophical Writings of Peirce*, New York: Dover Publications.

Perry, Chris, Krishna Chhatralia, Dom Damesick, Sylvie Hobden, and Leanora Volpe (2015), *Behavioral Insights in Health Care: Nudging to Reduce Inefficiency and Waste*, London: The Health Foundation.

Pilkey, Orrin H., and Linda Pilkey-Jarvis (2007), *Useless Arithmetic: Why Environmental Scientists Can't Predict the Future*, New York: Columbia University Press.

Pita, James, Manish Jain, Milind Tambe, Fernando Oróñez, and Sarit Kraus (2010), "Robust Solutions to Stackelberg Games: Addressing Bounded Rationality and Limited Observations in Human Cognition," *Artificial Intelligence*, 174 (150): 1142–1171.

Plumer, Brad, and Coral Davenport (2017), "E.P.A. to Give Dissenters a Voice on Climate, No Matter the Consensus," *New York Times*, Climate, A12, July 1. https://www.nytimes.com/2017/06/30/climate/scott-pruitt-climate-change-red-team.html

Political Science Program (2002), *The Empirical Impliciations of Theoretical Models (EITM) Workshop Report*, Washington, D.C.: National Science Foundation.

Popper, Steven W., James Griffin, Claude Berrebi, Thomas Light, and Endy Y. Min (2010), *Natural Gas and Israel's Energy Future: Near-Term Decisions from a Strategic Perspective*, Santa Monica, Calif.: Rand Corporation.

Post, Jerrold M., ed. (2008), *The Psychological Assessment of Political Leaders*, Ann Arbor: University of Michigan Press.

Pournelle, Phillip (2016), "MORS Wargaming Workshop," *Phalanx*, 49 (4), December.

President's Information Technology Advisory Committee (2005), *Computational Science: Ensuring America's Competitiveness*, Arlington, Virg.: National Coordination Office for Information Technology Research and Development.

Pruyt, Erik, and Tushith Islam (2015), "On Generating and Exploring the Behavior Space of Complex Models," *System Dynamics Review*, 31 (4), 220–249.

Pruyt, Erik, and Jan H. Kwakkel (2014), "Radicalization Under Deep Uncertainty: A Multi-Model Exploration of Activism, Extremism, and Terrorism," *System Dynamics Review*, 30 (1–2), 1–28.

Quade, Edward S. (1968), "Pitfalls and Limitations," in *Systems Analysis and Policy Planning: Applications to Defense*, edited by Edward S. Quade and Wayne I. Boucher, New York: Elsevier, 345–364.

Quade, Edward S., and Wayne I. Boucher, eds. (1968), *Systems Analysis and Policy Planning: Applications for Defense*, New York: Elsevier Science Publishers.

Quinlan, Philip T. (2003), "Visual Feature Integration Theory: Past, Present, and Future," *Psychological Bulletin*, 129 (5), 643–673.

Rahimian, M. Amoin, and Ali Jadbabaie (2016), "Bayesian Heuristics for Group Decisions," https://arxiv.org/abs/1611.01006 (accessed January 27, 2018).

Rahmandad, Hazhir, and John D. Sterman (2008), "Heterogeneity and Network Structure in the Dynamics of Diffusion: Comparing Agent-Based and Differential Equation Models," *Management Science*, 54 (5), 998–1014.

Read, Stephen J., Benjamin J. Smith, Vitaliya Droutman, and Lynn C. Miller (2017), "Virtual Personalities: Using Computational Modeling to Understand Within-Person Variability," *Journal of Research and Personality*, 69, 237–249.

Reiss, Julian, and Jan Sprinter (2017), "Scientific Objectivity," in *The Stanford Encyclopedia of Philosophy (Spring 2017 Edition)*, edited by Edward N. Zalta, Palo Alto, Calif.: Metaphysics Research Lab, Stanford University.

Rosenhead, Jonathan, and John Mingers, eds. (2002), *Rational Analysis for a Problematic World Revisited: Problem Structuring Methods for Complexity, Uncertainty, and Conflict*, 2nd ed., New York: John Wiley & Sons.

Rothenberg, Jeff (1989), "Tutorial: Artificial Intelligence and Simulation," in *Proceedings of the 1989 Winter Simulation Conference*, edited by E. A. MacNair, K. J. Musselman, and P. Heidelberger, IEEE, 33–39.

Rothenberg, Jeff, and Sanjai Narain (1994), *The RAND Advanced Simulation Language Project's Declarative Modeling Formalism (DMOD)*, Santa Monica, Calif.: RAND Corporation.

Rouse, William B. (2015), *Modeling and Visualization of Complex Systems and Enterprises*, Hoboken, N.J.: John Wiley & Sons.

Rouse, William B., and Kenneth R. Boff (2005), *Organizational Simulation*, Wiley-Interscience.

Ryan, Regina (2014), "Visualization for Sociocultural Understanding," in *Sociocultural Behavior Sensemaking: State of the Art in Understanding the Operational Environment*, edited by Jill D. Egeth, Gary L. Klein, and Dylan Schmorrow, McLean, Virg.: MITRE, 51–86.

Sambanis, Nicholas (2004), "Using Case Studies to Expand Economic Models of Civil War," *Perspectives on Politics*, 2 (02), 259–279.

Sanfilippo, Antonio, Eric Bell, and Courtney T. Corley (2014), "Current Trends in the Detection of Sociocultural Signatures: Data-Driven Models," in *Sociocultural Behavior Sensemaking: State of the Art in Understanding the Operational Environment*, edited by Jill D. Egeth, Gary Klein, and Dylan Schmorrow, McLean, Virg.: MITRE, 147–172.

Sargent, Robert G. (1984), "Verification and Validation of Simulation Models," in *Simulation and Model-Based Methodologies: An Integrative View*, edited by Tuncer I. Ören, Bernard P. Zeigler, and Maurice S. Elzas, Heidelberg: Springer-Verlag, 537–555.

——— (2010), "A Perspective on Modeling, Data, and Knowledge," in *Unifying Social Frameworks*, edited by the National Research Council, Washington, D.C.: National Academies Press

Schelling, Thomas C. (1971), "Dynamic Models of Segregation," *Journal of Mathematical Sociology*, 1, 143–186.

Schrodt, Philip A. (2013), "Seven Deadly Sins of Contemporary Quantitative Political Analysis," *Journal of Peace Research*, 51 (2), 283–300.

Schwabe, William L. (1994), *An Introduction to Analytic Gaming*, Santa Monica, Calif.: RAND Corporation, P-7864.

Simon, Herbert (1957), "A Behavioral Model of Rational Choice," in *Models of Man: Social and Rational,* New York: Wiley, 198.

——— (1990), "Prediction and Prescription in Systems Modeling," *Operations Research*, 38 (1), 7–14.

——— (1996), *The Sciences of the Artificial*, 3rd ed., Cambridge, Mass.: MIT Press.

Sliva, Amy (2014), "Methods and Tools to Analyze Responding to Counteracting and Utilizing Sociocultural Behaviors," in *Sociocultural Behavior Sensemaking: State of the Art in Understanding the Operational Environment*, edited by Jill D. Egeth, Gary L. Klein, and Dylan Schmorrow, McLean, Virg.: MITRE, 385–406.

Steeb, Randall, John Matsumura, Thomas J. Herbert, John Gordon IV, and William W. Horn (2011), *Perspectives on the Battle of Wanat: Challenges Facing Small Unit Operations in Afghanistan*, Santa Monica, Calif.: RAND Corporation, OP-329/1-A.

Sterman, John D. (2000), *Business Dynamics: Systems Thinking and Modeling for a Complex World*, Boston: McGraw-Hill.

Stokes, Donald E. (1997), *Pasteur's Quadrant: Basic Science and Technological Innovation*, Washington, D.C.: Brookings Institution Press.

Sunstein, Cass R. (2014), *Why Nudge?: The Politics of Libertarian Paternalism (the Storrs Lectures Series)*, New Haven, Conn.: Yale University Press.

Swedberg, Richard (2014), *The Art of Social Theory*, Princeton, N.J.: Princeton University Press.

Szyperski, Clemens (2002), *Component Software: Beyond Object-Oriented Programming*, 2nd ed., New York: Addison-Wesley.

Taylor, Simon J. E., Azman Kahn, Katherine L. Morse, Andreas Tolk, Levent Yilmaz, Justyna Zander, and Pieter J. Mosterman (2015), "Grand Challenges for Modeling and Simulation: Simulation Everywhere—From Cyberinfrastructure to Clouds to Citizens," *Simulation*, 91, 648–655.

Tesfatsion, Leigh (2018), "Electric Power Markets in Transition: Agent-Based Modeling Tools for Transactive Energy Support," in *Handbook of Computational Economics 4: Heterogeneous Agent Models*, edited by C. Hommes, and B. LeBaron, Amsterdam: Elsevier.

Thacker, Ben H., Scott W. Doubling, Francois M. Hersez, Marc C. Anderson, Jason E. Pepin, and Edward A. Rodriguez (2004), *Concepts of Model Verification and Validation*, LA-14167-MS, Los Alamos, N.M.: Los Alamos National Laboratory.

Thaler, Richard H., and Cass R. Sunstein (2009), *Nudge: Improving Decisions About Health, Wealth, and Happiness*, New York: Penguin Books.

Tolk, Andreas (2012a), "Chapter 14: Verification and Validation," in *Engineering Principles of Combat Modeling and Distributed Simulation*, edited by Andreas Tolk, Hoboken, N.J.: Wiley, 263–294.

Tolk, Andreas, ed. (2012b), *Engineering Principles of Combat Modeling and Distributed Simulation*, Hoboken, N.J.: Wiley.

Tolk, Andreas, Saikou Diallo, Jose J. Padilla, and Heber Herencia-Zapana (2013), "Reference Modeling in Support of M&S—Foundations and Applications," *Journal of Simulation*, 7, 69–82.

Turnley, Jessica Glicken (2011), "Assessing the 'Goodness' of Computational Social Models," in *Challenges in Computational Social Modeling and Simulation for National Security Decision-Making*, edited by Laura A. McNamara, Timothy G. Trucano, and Charles Gieseler, Fort Belvoir, Virg.: Defense Threat Reduction Agency, Advanced Systems and Concept Office, 241–255.

Uhrmacher, Adelinde, Mathias Röhl, and Beth Kulick (2002), "The Role of Reflection in Simulating and Testing Agents: An Exploration Based on the Simulation System James," *Applied Artificial Intelligence*, 16 (9–10), 795–811.

Uhrmacher, Adelinde M., Sally Brailsford, Jason Liu, Markus Rabe, and Andreas Tolk, (2016), "Panel: Reproducible Research in Discrete Event Simulation—A Must or Rather a Maybe?," in *2016 Winter Simulation Conference*, edited by T.M.K. Roeder et al., IEEE, 1301–1315.

Uhrmacher, Adelinde, and Bernard P. Zeigler (1996), "Variable Structure Models in Object-Oriented Simulation," *International Journal of General Systems*, 24 (4), 359–375.

U.S. General Accountability Office (1989), *ICBM Modernization: Availability Problems and Flight Test Delays in Peacekeeper Program*, Washington, D.C.: GPO.

Waltzman, Rand (2017), "The Weaponization of Information: The Need for Cognitive Security," testimony, Santa Monica, Calif.: RAND Corporation, CT-473.

Weinberg, Steven (1994), *Dreams of a Final Theory: The Scientist's Search for the Ultimate Laws of Nature*, New York: Vintage.

West, Geoffrey (2017), *Scale: The Universal Laws of Growth, Innovation, Sustainability, and the Pace of Life in Organisms, Cities, Economies, and Companies*, New York: Penguin Press.

Whipple, Chris G. (2007), *Models in Environmental Regulatory Decision Making*, Washington, D.C.: National Academics Press.

Wilensky, Uri, and William Rand (2007), "Making Models Match: Replicating an Agent-Based Model," *Journal of Artificial Societies and Social Simulation*, 10(4).

Yilmaz, Levent (2006a), "A Strategy for Improving Dynamic Composability: Ontology-Driven Introspective Agent Architectures," *Systemics, Cybernetics, and Informatics*, 5(5), 1–9.

——— (2006b), "Validation and Verification of Social Processes Within Agent-Based Computational Models," *Computational and Mathematical Organization Theory*, 12, 283–312.

——— (2012), "Reproducibility in M&S Research: Issues, Strategies, and Implications for Model Development Environments," *Journal of Experimental and Theoretical Artificial Intelligence*, 24 (4), 457–474.

Yilmaz, Levent, Alvin Lim, Simon Bowen, and Tuncer Ören (2007), "Requirements and Design Principles for Multisimulation with Multiresolution Multistage Models," *Winter Simulation Conference 2007*, IEEE, 823–832.

Yilmaz, Levent, and Tuncer I. Ören (2006), "Prospective Issues in Simulation Model Composability: Basic Concepts to Advance Theory, Methodology, and Technology," *MSIAC's M&S Journal Online*, 2.

——— (2009), *Agent-Directed Simulation and Systems Engineering*, Weinheim: Wiley-VCH.

——— (2013), "Toward Replicability-Aware Modeling and Simulation: Changing the Conduct of M&S in the Information Age," in *Ontology, Epistemology, and Teleology for Modeling and Simulation*, edited by Levent Yilmaz and Tuncer I. Ören, Berlin and Heidelberg: Springer, 207–226.

Yost, Beth (2014), "Interactive Data Visualization for Mitigation Planning: Comparing and Contrasting Options," in *Sociocultural Behavior Sensemaking: State of the Art in Understanding the Operational Environment*, edited by Jill D. Egeth, G. Klein, and Dylan Schmorrow, McLean, Virg.: MITRE, 407–428.

Youngblood, Simone M., Dale K. Pace, Peter L. Eirich, Donna M. Gregg, and James E. Coolahan (2000), "Simulation Verification, Validation, and Accreditation," *Johns Hopkins Applied Physics Laboratory*, 21 (3), 359–367.

Youngman, Paul A., and Mirsad Hadzikadic, eds. (2014), *Complexity and the Human Experience: Modeling Complexity in the Humanities and Social Sciences*, Boca Raton, Fla.: CRC Press, Taylor & Francis Group.

Zacharias, Greg L., Jean MacMillan, and Susan B. Van Hemel, eds. (2008), *Behavioral Modeling and Simulation: From Individuals to Societies*, Washington, D.C.: National Academies Press.

Zak, Paul J. (2012), *The Moral Molecule: The Source of Love and Prosperity*, New York: Dutton.

Zech, Steven T., and Michael Gabbay (2016), "Social Network Analysis in the Study of Terrorism and Insurgency: From Organization to Politics," *Omtermatopma; Studies Review*, 18 (2), 214–243.

Zeigler, Bernard (1984), *Multifaceted Modelling and Discrete Event Simulation*, Ontario, Calif.: Academic Press.

Zeigler, Bernard, Herbert Praenhofer, and Tag Gon Kim (2000), *Theory of Modeling and Simulation, 2nd Edition: Integrating Discrete Event and Continuous Complex Systems*, San Diego, Calif.: John Wiley & Sons.

Zeigler, Bernard P. (1998), "A Framework for Modeling and Simulation," in *Applied Modeling and Simulation: An Integrated Approach to Development and Operations*, edited by David S. Cloud and Larry B. Rainey, New York: McGraw Hill, 67–103.

Zeigler, Bernard P., and Phillip E. Hammond (2007), *Modeling and Simulation-Based Data Engineering: Introducing Pragmatics into Ontologies for Information Exchange*, New York: Academic Press.

Zeuch, Richard, Taghi Khoshgoftaar, and Randall Wald (2015), "Intrusion Detection and Big Heterogeneous Data: A Survey," *Journal of Big Data*, 2 (1), 1.

Zhang, Haifeng, Yevgeniy Vorobeychik, Joshua Letchford, and Kran Lakkaraju (2016), "Data-Driven Agent-Based Modeling with Application to Rooftop Solar Adoption," *Autonomous Agents and Multi-Agent Systems,* 30 (6), 1023–1049.

Zyda, Michael (2007), "Creating a Science of Games," *Communications-ACM*, 50 (7), 26.